T0214563

Lecture Notes in Computer Science 11042

Commenced Publication in 1973
Founding and Former Series Editors:
Gerhard Goos, Juris Hartmanis, and Jan van Leeuwen

More information about this series at http://www.springer.com/series/7412

Danail Stoyanov · Zeike Taylor
Stephen Aylward · João Manuel R. S. Tavares
Yiming Xiao · Amber Simpson et al. (Eds.)

Simulation, Image Processing, and Ultrasound Systems for Assisted Diagnosis and Navigation

International Workshops, POCUS 2018, BIVPCS 2018,
CuRIOUS 2018, and CPM 2018
Held in Conjunction with MICCAI 2018
Granada, Spain, September 16–20, 2018
Proceedings

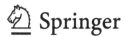 Springer

Editors
Danail Stoyanov
University College London
London, UK

Zeike Taylor
University of Leeds
Leeds, UK

Stephen Aylward ⓘ
Kitware Inc.
Carrboro, NC, USA

João Manuel R. S. Tavares ⓘ
University of Porto
Porto, Portugal

Yiming Xiao ⓘ
Robarts Research Institute
Western University
London, ON, Canada

Amber Simpson ⓘ
Memorial Sloan Kettering Cancer Center
New York, NY, USA

Additional Workshop Editors *see next page*

ISSN 0302-9743   ISSN 1611-3349   (electronic)
Lecture Notes in Computer Science
ISBN 978-3-030-01044-7   ISBN 978-3-030-01045-4   (eBook)
https://doi.org/10.1007/978-3-030-01045-4

Library of Congress Control Number: 2018955279

LNCS Sublibrary: SL6 – Image Processing, Computer Vision, Pattern Recognition, and Graphics

This Springer imprint is published by the registered company Springer Nature Switzerland AG
The registered company address is: Gewerbestrasse 11, 6330 Cham, Switzerland

Additional Workshop Editors

Tutorial and Educational Chair

Anne Martel
University of Toronto
Toronto, ON
Canada

Workshop and Challenge Co-chair

Lena Maier-Hein
German Cancer Research Center (DKFZ)
Heidelberg
Germany

International Workshop on Bio-Imaging and Visualization for Patient-Customized Simulations, BIVPCS 2018

Shuo Li
University of Western Ontario
London, ON
Canada

International Workshop on Correction of Brainshift with Intra-Operative Ultrasound, CuRIOUS 2018

Hassan Rivaz
Concordia University
Montréal, QC
Canada

Matthieu Chabanas
Grenoble Institute of Technology
Grenoble
France

Ingerid Reinertsen
SINTEF Health Research
Trondheim
Norway

International Workshop on Computational Precision Medicine, CPM 2018

Keyvan Farahani
National Cancer Institute
Bethesda, MD
USA

POCUS 2018 Preface

For the full potential of point-of-care ultrasound (POCUS) to be realized, POCUS systems must be approached as if they were new diagnostic modalities, not simply inexpensive, portable ultrasound image systems. Building on the highly successful MICCAI 2017 POCUS Workshop, this MICCAI 2018 workshop dedicated to the research and clinical evaluations of the technologies specific to POCUS. POCUS involves automated data analyses, rugged hardware, and specialized interfaces to guide novice users to properly place and manipulate an ultrasound probe and interpret the returned ultrasound data. In particular, the output of a POCUS system should typically be quantitative measures and easy-to-understand reformulations of the acquired data, not b-mode images; it should be assumed that the expertise needed to interpret b-mode images will not be readily available at the points of care. Image analysis algorithms as well as tracking and systems engineering are essential to POCUS applications. Example applications include detection of intra-abdominal bleeding by emergency medical services (EMS) personnel for patient triage at the scene of an accident, diagnosis of increased intra-cranial pressure by medics using computer-assisted measurement of optic nerve sheath diameter, and monitoring of liver tissue health in the homes of at-risk patients. At the workshop, attendees learned from leaders in POCUS research via oral presentations as well as via numerous live demonstrations.

September 2018

Stephen Aylward
Emad Boctor
Gabor Fitchinger

BIVPCS 2018 Preface

Imaging and visualization are among the most dynamic and innovative areas of research of the past few decades. Justification of this activity arises from the requirements of important practical applications such as the visualization of computational data, the processing of medical images for assisting medical diagnosis and intervention, and the 3D geometry reconstruction and processing for computer simulations. Currently, owing to the development of more powerful hardware resources, mathematical and physical methods, investigators have been incorporating advanced computational techniques to derive sophisticated methodologies that can better enable the solution of the problems encountered. Consequent to these efforts, any effective methodologies have been proposed, validated, and some of them have already been integrated into commercial software for computer simulations. The main goal of this MICCAI workshop on "Bio-Imaging and Visualization for Patient-Customized Simulations" is to provide a platform for communication among specialists from complementary fields such as signal and image processing, mechanics, computational vision, mathematics, physics, informatics, computer graphics, bio-medical practice, psychology and industry. Another important objective of this MICCAI workshop is to establish a viable connection between software developers, specialist researchers, and applied end-users from diverse fields related to signal processing, imaging, visualization, biomechanics and simulation. This book contains the full papers presented at the MICCAI 2018 workshop on "Bio-Imaging and Visualization for Patient-Customized Simulations" (MWBIVPCS 2018), which was organized under the auspices of the 21st International Conference on Medical Image Computing and Computer-Assisted Intervention 2018 that was held in Granada, Spain, during September 16–20, 2018. MWBIVPCS 2018 brought together researchers representing several fields, such as biomechanics, engineering, medicine, mathematics, physics, and statistics. The works included in this book present and discuss new trends in those fields, using several methods and techniques, including convolutional neural networks, similarity metrics, atlas, level-set, deformable models, GPGPU programming, sparse annotation, and sensors calibration, in order to address more efficiently different and timely applications involving signal and image acquisition, image processing and analysis, image visualization, image segmentation, image reconstruction, image fusion, computer simulation, image based modelling, ray tracing, virtual reality, image-based diagnosis, surgery planning and simulation, and therapy planning. The editors wish to thank all the MWBIVPCS 2018 authors and members of the Program Committee for sharing their expertise, and also the MICCAI Society for having hosted and supported the workshop within MICCAI 2018.

September 2018

João Manuel R. S. Tavares
Shuo Li

CuRIOUS 2018 Preface

Radical brain tumor resection can effectively improve the patient's survival. However, resection quality and safety can often be heavily affected by intra-operative brain tissue shift due to factors such as gravity, drug administration, intracranial pressure change, and tissue removal. Such tissue shift can displace the surgical target and vital structures (e.g., blood vessels) shown in pre-operative images while these displacements may not be directly visible in the surgeon's field of view. Intra-operative ultrasound (iUS) is a robust and relatively inexpensive technique to track intra-operative tissue shift. To update pre-surgical plans with this information, accurate and robust image registration algorithms are needed in order to relate pre-surgical magnetic resonance imaging (MRI) to iUS images. Despite the great progress so far, medical image registration techniques are still not in routine clinical use in neurosurgery to directly benefit patients with brain tumors. The MICCAI Challenge 2018 for Correction of Brain Shift with Intra-Operative Ultrasound (CuRIOUS) offered a snapshot of the state-of-the-art progress in the field through extended discussions, and provided researchers with an opportunity to characterize their image registration methods on a newly released standardized dataset of iUS-guided brain tumor resection.

September 2018

Ingerid Reinertsen
Hassan Rivaz
Yiming Xiao
Matthieu Chabanas

CPM 2018 Preface

On September 16, 2018, the Workshop and Challenges in Computational Precision Medicine were held in Granada, Spain, in conjunction with the 21st International Conference on Medical Image Computing and Computer-Assisted Intervention (MICCAI). This year's edition featured a workshop held in the morning followed by the presentation of challenges in the afternoon.

The workshop featured topics in quantitative imaging data science, artificial intelligence and machine learning, and applications of radiomics in cancer diagnosis and therapy. Invited speakers included prominent members of the community: Drs. J. Kalpathy-Cramer (Massachusetts General Hospital), C. Davatzikos (University of Pennsylvania), A. Simpson (Memorial Sloan Kettering Cancer Center), D. Fuller (MD Anderson), K. Yan, R. Summers (National Cancer Institutes), Anne Martel (University of Toronto), and J. Liu (National Institutes of Health).

Members of the MICCAI community were encouraged to participate in four challenges this year:

1. Pancreatic Cancer Survival Prediction Challenge
2. Combined Imaging and Digital Pathology Brain Tumor Classification Challenge
3. Digital Pathology Nuclei Segmentation Challenge
4. Radiomics Stratifiers in Oropharynx Challenge

In response to the call for challenge participants, 239 participants registered for the Pancreatic Cancer Survival Prediction Challenge, 203 participants registered for the Combined Imaging and Digital Pathology Brain Tumor Classification Challenge, and 261 participants registered for the Digital Pathology Nuclei Segmentation Challenge. The top three winners of each challenge gave brief presentations of their algorithms during the challenge sessions.

This volume of papers represents the top two submissions from the Pancreatic Cancer Survival Prediction Challenge. Participants were provided with segmented CT scans and limited clinical data. The task was to predict overall survival. The training phase of the challenge started on May 15, 2018, and the test phase started on August 1, 2018, and concluded on August 15, 2018.

We thank the MICCAI Program Committee for the opportunity to host the CPM workshop and challenges again this year. Our thanks also go out to our workshop presenters and to all of the teams that participated in the challenges.

August 2018

Spyridon Bakas
Hesham El Halawani
Keyvan Farahani
John Freymann
David Fuller
Jayashree Kalpathy-Cramer
Justin Kirby
Tahsin Kurc
Joel Saltz
Amber Simpson

Organization

POCUS 2018 Organizing Committee

Stephen Aylward	Kitware, USA
Emad Boctor	Johns Hopkins University, USA
Gabor Fitchinger	Queens University, Canada

BIVPCS 2018 Organizing Committee

João Manuel R. S. Tavares	University of Porto, Portugal
Shuo Li	University of Western Ontario, Canada

CuRIOUS 2018 Organizing Committee

Ingerid Reinertsen	SINTEF, Norway
Hassan Rivaz	Concordia University, Canada
Yiming Xiao	Western University, Canada
Matthieu Chabanas	University of Grenoble Alpes, Grenoble Institute of Technology, France

CPM 2018 Organizing Committee

Spyridon Bakas	University of Pennsylvania, USA
Hesham El Halawani	MD Anderson Cancer Center, USA
Keyvan Farahani	National Cancer Institute, USA
John Freymann	Leidos Biomedical Research, USA
David Fuller	MD Anderson Cancer Center, USA
Jayashree Kalpathy-Cramer	MGH Harvard, USA
Justin Kirby	Leidos Biomedical Research, USA
Tahsin Kurc	Stony Brook Cancer Center, USA
Joel Saltz	Stony Brook Cancer Center, USA
Amber Simpson	Memorial Sloan Kettering Cancer Center, USA

Contents

International Workshop on Computational Precision Medicine, CPM 2018

International Workshop
on Point-of-Care Ultrasound,
POCUS 2018

Robust Photoacoustic Beamforming Using Dense Convolutional Neural Networks

Emran Mohammad Abu Anas[1(✉)], Haichong K. Zhang[1], Chloé Audigier[2], and Emad M. Boctor[1,2]

[1] Electrical and Computer Engineering, Johns Hopkins University,
Baltimore, MD, USA
eanas1@jhmi.edu

[2] Radiology and Radiological Science, Johns Hopkins University,
Baltimore, MD, USA

Abstract. Photoacoustic (PA) is a promising technology for imaging of endogenous tissue chromophores and exogenous contrast agents in a wide range of clinical applications. The imaging technique is based on excitation of a tissue sample using short light pulse, followed by acquisition of the resultant acoustic signal using an ultrasound (US) transducer. To reconstruct an image of the tissue from the received US signals, the most common approach is to use the delay-and-sum (DAS) beamforming technique that assumes a wave propagation with a constant speed of sound. Unfortunately, such assumption often leads to artifacts such as sidelobes and tissue aberration; in addition, the image resolution is degraded. With an aim to improve the PA image reconstruction, in this work, we propose a deep convolutional neural networks-based beamforming approach that uses a set of densely connected convolutional layers with dilated convolution at higher layers. To train the network, we use simulated images with various sizes and contrasts of target objects, and subsequently simulating the PA effect to obtain the raw US signals at an US transducer. We test the network on an independent set of 1,500 simulated images and we achieve a mean peak-to-signal-ratio of 38.7 dB between the estimated and reference images. In addition, a comparison of our approach with the DAS beamforming technique indicates a statistical significant improvement of the proposed technique.

Keywords: Photoacoustic · Beamforming · Delay-and-sum
Convolutional neural networks · Dense convolution
Dilated convolution

1 Introduction

Photoacoustic (PA) is considered as a hybrid imaging modality that combines optical and ultrasound (US) imaging techniques. The underlying physics of this

© Springer Nature Switzerland AG 2018
D. Stoyanov et al. (Eds.): POCUS 2018/BIVPCS 2018/CuRIOUS 2018/CPM 2018,
LNCS 11042, pp. 3–11, 2018.
https://doi.org/10.1007/978-3-030-01045-4_1

imaging technology is based on the PA effect that refers to the phenomenon of generation of acoustic waves following a short light pulse absorption in a soft-tissue sample. To exploit the PA effect and enable imaging of that soft-tissue, a light source (laser or light emitting diode) is employed to excite the soft-tissue, and simultaneously an US transducer is used to collect the instantaneously generated acoustic signal. In contrast to the acoustic properties-based pure US imaging technique, the PA imaging modality provides functional information (e.g., hemoglobin in blood and melanin in skin) of the anatomy. Based on this fact, the key applications of PA imaging have been found in detection of ischemic stroke, breast cancer or skin melanomas [3,7]. In addition to tissue chromophores, the PA technique has shown its ability to image exogenous contrast agents in a number of clinical applications including molecular imaging and prostate cancer detection [1,18].

The most common approach to reconstruct a PA image from the received US signal (channel data) is the delay-and-sum (DAS) beamforming technique due to its simple implementation and real-time capability. In short, the output of the DAS method is obtained by averaging the weighted and delayed versions of the received US signals. The delay calculation is based on an assumption of an US wave propagation with a constant speed of sound (SoS), therefore, it compromises the image quality of a DAS beamformer [5]. To improve the beamforming with PA imaging, a significant number of works have been reported using, for example, minimum variance [11], coherence factor [13], short-lag spatial coherence beamforming [4], adaptive beamforming [15] and double-stage delay-multiply-and-sum beamforming [12]. Though these approaches have shown their potential to improve the beamforming, they are less robust to tackle the SoS variation in different applications.

In the recent years, deep learning based approaches have demonstrated their promising performance compared to the previous state-of-the-art image processing approaches in almost all areas of computer vision. In addition to vision recognition, deep neural techniques have been successfully applied for beamforming [2,9,10,14] of US signal. Luchies et al. [9,10] presented deep neural networks for US beamforming from the raw channel data. However, their proposed network is based on fully connected layers that are prone to overfit the network parameters. Nair et al. [14] recently proposed a deep convolutional neural networks (CNN)-based image transformation approach to map the channel data to US images. In fact, their output US image is a binary segmentation map instead of an intensity image, therefore, it does not preserve the relative contrast among the target objects that is considered quite important in functional PA imaging.

In this work, we propose a deep CNN-based approach to reconstruct a PA image from the raw US signals. Unlike the techniques in [9,10], we use fully convolutional networks for the beamforming of the US signals that reduces the problem of overfitting the network parameters. In addition, our proposed network maps the channel data to an intensity image that keeps the relative contrast among the target objects. The network consists of a set of densely connected convolutional layers [6] that have shown their effectiveness to eliminate the gradient vanishing problem during training. Furthermore, we exploit dilated convolution [17] at higher layers in our architecture to allow feature extraction without loss of resolution. The training of the network is based on simulation experiments that consist of simulated target objects in different SoS environments. Such a variation in SoS during training makes the proposed network less sensitive to SoS changes when mapping the channel data to a PA image.

2   Methods

Figure 1(a) shows the architecture of our proposed deep CNN that maps an input channel data to an output PA image. Note that the channel data refers to the pre-beamformed RF data in this whole work. The sizes of the input and output images of the network are 384×128. The network consists of five dense blocks representing convolution at five different scales. In each dense block, there are two densely connected convolutional layers with 16 feature maps in each layer. The size of all of the convolutional kernels is 9×9 and each convolution is followed by rectified linear unit (ReLU). The key principle of dense convolution is using all of the previous features at its input, therefore, the features are propagated more effectively, subsequently, the vanishing gradient problem is eliminated [6]. In addition to dense convolution, we use dilated convolution [17] at higher layers of our architecture to overcome the problem of losing resolution at those layers. We set the dilation factors for the dense block 1 to 5 as 1, 2, 4, 8 and 16, respectively (Fig. 1(a)). The dilated convolution is a special convolution that

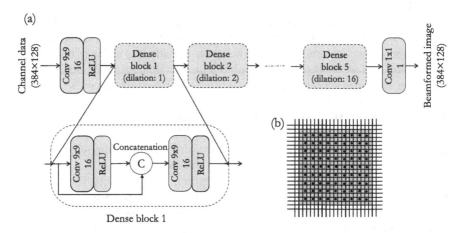

Fig. 1. The proposed beamforming approach. (a) The neural network architecture to map the channel data to a PA image. The network consists of five dense blocks, where each dense block consists of two densely connected convolutional layers followed by ReLU. The difference among five dense blocks lies in the amount of dilation factor. (b) Effect of dilation on the effective receptive field size. A dilated convolution of a kernel size of 9×9 with a dilation factor of 2 indicates an effective receptive field size of 19×19.

allows the convolution operation without decreasing the resolution of the feature maps but using the same number of convolutional kernel parameters. Figure 1(b) shows an example of a dilated convolution for a kernel size of 9×9 with a dilation factor of 2 that represents an effective receptive field size of 19×19. A successive increase in the dilation factor across layer 1 to 5, therefore, indicates a successively greater effective receptive field size. At the end of the network, we perform 1×1 convolution to predict an output image from the generated feature maps. The loss function of the network consists of the mean square losses between the predicted and target images.

3   Experiments and Training

3.1   Experiments and Materials

We perform simulation experiments to train, validate and test the proposed network. Each experiment consists of a number of simulated 2D target objects with different sizes and contrasts. In this work, we consider only circular target objects because their shapes are highly similar to those of the blood vessels in 2D planes, where most of the PA applications have been reported. In each simulation, we randomly choose the total number (between 1 and 6 inclusive) of target objects. In addition, the SoS of the background as well as of the targets is set as constant for each experiment and it is randomly chosen in the range of 1450–1550 m/s. Each target is modeled by a Gaussian function, where position of the target and its peak intensity (corresponding to contrast) are randomly chosen. The size of the target is controlled by the standard deviation of the Gaussian function, and it is also chosen randomly within a range of 0.2–1.0 mm. We have performed a total of 5,000 simulations to obtain the simulated images. For each image, we generate the channel data considering a linear transducer with 128 elements at the top of the simulated image (simulating PA effect) using the k-Wave simulation toolbox [16]. In addition, we have introduced white noise with Gaussian distribution on the channel data to allow the proposed network to be robust against the noise. The variance of the noise is randomly chosen as a number that is always less than the power of the signal in each experiment. Figure 2 shows an example of simulated image and corresponding channel data with 4 target objects with different sizes and contrasts.

We divide all of our images into three groups to constitute the training, validation and test sets. The images are distributed independently as 60% vs 10% vs 30% for the training, validation and test sets, respectively. Therefore, the total number of training, validation and test images are 3,000, 500 and 1,500, respectively, in this work.

3.2   Training and Validation

We use the TensorFlow library (Google, Mountain View, CA) with Adam [8] optimization technique to train the proposed network based on the training set.

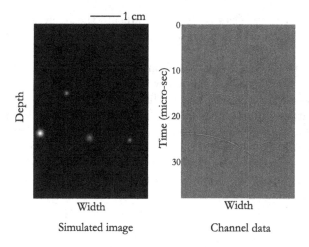

Fig. 2. An example of simulated PA image with 4 targets (left figure). We can notice the variation of sizes and contrasts among the targets. From the simulated image, we use the k-Wave simulation toolbox [16] to obtain the channel data (right figure).

A total of 8,000 epochs is used to optimize the network parameters in our GPU (NVIDIA GeForce GTX 1080 Ti with 11 GB RAM) with a mini-batch size of 16. The initial learning rate is set to 10^{-3} and there is an exponential decay of the learning rate after each successive 2,000 epochs with a decay factor of 0.1.

While the training set is used to optimize the network parameters, the validation set in our work is used to fix the hyper-parameters of our network including the size of the convolutional kernel (9×9), the number of convolutional layers (2) in each dense block, the number of feature maps (16) in each dense convolution and the initial learning rate (10^{-3}) in the Adam optimization.

4 Evaluation and Results

4.1 Evaluation

To evaluate the proposed beamforming approach using the test set, we use the peak-signal-to-noise-ratio (PSNR) that is based on the mean square losses between the estimated and reference images in decibels (dB) as:

$$\text{PSNR} = 20 \log_{10}\left(\frac{I_{\max}}{\sqrt{MSE}}\right) \quad \text{dB},\tag{1}$$

where,

$$MSE = \frac{1}{MN} \sum_{m=0}^{M-1} \sum_{n=0}^{N-1} \left(I_{\text{ref}}(m,n) - I_{\text{est}}(m,n)\right)^2.$$

Here, I_{ref} and I_{est} (both sizes of $M \times N$) indicate the reference and estimated images, respectively; and I_{max} represents the maximum intensity in the reference image.

In addition to the evaluation based on PSNR, we investigate the sensitivity of the proposed beamforming technique with respect to SoS variation across different test images. For this purpose, we divide the whole range (1450–1550 m/s) of SoS distribution in the test set into 10 different non-overlapping sets, followed by computation of the PSNR in that non-overlapping region. Furthermore, we compare our approach with widely accepted DAS beamforming technique. Note that the SoS parameter in the DAS method is set to 1500 m/s in this comparison. Finally, we report the computation time of the proposed method in GPU to check its real-time capability.

4.2   Results

Based on 1,500 test images, we achieve a PSNR of 38.7 ± 4.3 dB compared to that of 30.5 ± 2.4 dB for the DAS technique. A student t-test is performed to determine the statistical significance between the obtained results of these two techniques, and the obtained p-value ≪ 0.01 indicates the superiority of the proposed method.

Figures 3(a–c) present a qualitative comparison among reference, DAS- and our CNN-beamformed images, respectively. In this particular example, we observe the distortion of the circular targets (marked by arrows) by the DAS beamforming technique. In contrast, the presented technique preserves the shapes and sizes of the targets. For a better visualization, we plot the PA intensity along a line (marked by dotted lines in Figs. 3(a–c)) in Fig. 3(d) and it indicates the promising performance of our proposed beamforming method, i.e., the width of the object is well preserved in our reconstruction.

Figure 3(e) shows a comparison between our and DAS methods in PSNR with respect to SoS variation based on the test set. As mentioned earlier, for a better interpretation of the sensitivity of the beamforming approaches, we divide the whole range (1450–1550 m/s) of SoS into 10 different non-overlapping sets, and we use the mean SoS of each set along the x-axis in this figure. The comparison between our and DAS beamforming techniques indicates less sensitivity of the DAS technique on the SoS variation in the test images. It is also interesting to note that the best performance of the DAS method is obtained for a SoS in the 1490–1500 m/s range. It is expected as this SoS is closer to the inherent SoS (1500 m/s) assumption in the DAS technique.

The run-time of the proposed CNN-based beamforming method is 18 ms in our GPU-based computer.

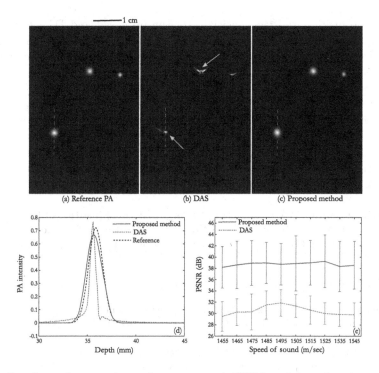

Fig. 3. Results and comparison of our proposed CNN-based beamforming method. (a–c) A comparison between DAS and our technique with respect to the reference PA image. The distortions in the targets are well visible in the DAS-beamformed image (marked by arrows). (d) The PA intensity variation along depth. This particular intensity variation corresponds to the dotted lines in (a–c). (e) Sensitivity of our and DAS methods with respect to SoS variation. For this figure, we divide the whole range of SoS (1450–1550 m/s) distribution in the test set into 10 different non-overlapping sets, and the x-axis represents the mean values of these sets. We can observe less sensitivity of our technique on SoS changes, in contrast, the DAS method shows its best performance at SoS near 1500 m/s.

5 Discussion and Conclusion

In this work, we have presented a deep CNN-based real-time beamforming approach to map the channel data to a PA image. Two notable modifications in the architecture are the incorporation of dense and dilated convolutions that lead to an improved training and a feature extraction without losing the resolution. The network has been trained using a set of simulation experiments with various contrasts and sizes of multiple targets. On the test set of 1,500 simulated images, we could obtain a mean PSNR of 38.7 dB.

A comparison of our result with that of the DAS beamforming method indicates a significant improvement achieved by the proposed technique. In addition, we have demonstrated how our method preserves the shapes and sizes of various targets in PA images (Figs. 3(a–d)).

We have investigated the sensitivity of the proposed and DAS beamforming methods on the SoS variation in test images. Since there is a inherent SoS assumption in the DAS method, it has shown its best performance at SoS near its SoS assumption. In contrast, our proposed beamforming technique has demonstrated less sensitivity to SoS changes in the test set (Fig. 3(e)).

Future works include training with non-circular targets, and testing on phantom and *in vivo* images. In addition, we aim to compare our method with neural networks-based beamforming approaches.

In conclusion, we have demonstrated the potential of the proposed CNN-based technique to beamform the channel data to a PA image in real-time while preserving the shapes and sizes of the targets.

Acknowledgements. We would like to thank the National Institute of Health (NIH) Brain Initiative (R24MH106083-03) and NIH National Institute of Biomedical Imaging and Bioengineering (R01EB01963) for funding this project.

References

1. Agarwal, A., et al.: Targeted gold nanorod contrast agent for prostate cancer detection by photoacoustic imaging. J. Appl. Phys. **102**(6), 064701 (2007)
2. Antholzer, S., Haltmeier, M., Schwab, J.: Deep learning for photoacoustic tomography from sparse data. arXiv preprint arXiv:1704.04587 (2017)
3. Beard, P.: Biomedical photoacoustic imaging. Interface Focus (2011). https://doi.org/10.1098/rsfs.2011.0028
4. Bell, M.A.L., Kuo, N., Song, D.Y., Boctor, E.M.: Short-lag spatial coherence beamforming of photoacoustic images for enhanced visualization of prostate brachytherapy seeds. Biomed. Optics Express **4**(10), 1964–1977 (2013)
5. Hoelen, C.G., de Mul, F.F.: Image reconstruction for photoacoustic scanning of tissue structures. Appl. Opt. **39**(31), 5872–5883 (2000)
6. Huang, G., Liu, Z., Weinberger, K.Q., van der Maaten, L.: Densely connected convolutional networks. In: Proceedings of the IEEE Conference on Computer Vision and Pattern Recognition, vol. 1, p. 3 (2017)
7. Kang, J., et al.: Validation of noninvasive photoacoustic measurements of sagittal sinus oxyhemoglobin saturation in hypoxic neonatal piglets. J. Appl. Physiol. (2018)
8. Kingma, D., Ba, J.: Adam: a method for stochastic optimization. arXiv preprint arXiv:1412.6980 (2014)
9. Luchies, A., Byram, B.: Deep neural networks for ultrasound beamforming. In: 2017 IEEE International Ultrasonics Symposium (IUS), pp. 1–4. IEEE (2017)
10. Luchies, A., Byram, B.: Suppressing off-axis scattering using deep neural networks. In: Medical Imaging 2018: Ultrasonic Imaging and Tomography, vol. 10580, p. 105800G. International Society for Optics and Photonics (2018)
11. Mozaffarzadeh, M., Mahloojifar, A., Orooji, M.: Medical photoacoustic beamforming using minimum variance-based delay multiply and sum. In: Digital Optical Technologies 2017, vol. 10335, p. 1033522. International Society for Optics and Photonics (2017)
12. Mozaffarzadeh, M., Mahloojifar, A., Orooji, M., Adabi, S., Nasiriavanaki, M.: Double-stage delay multiply and sum beamforming algorithm: application to linear-array photoacoustic imaging. IEEE Trans. Biomed. Eng. **65**(1), 31–42 (2018)

13. Mozaffarzadeh, M., Yan, Y., Mehrmohammadi, M., Makkiabadi, B.: Enhanced linear-array photoacoustic beamforming using modified coherence factor. J. Biomed. Opt. **23**(2), 026005 (2018)
14. Nair, A.A., Tran, T.D., Reiter, A., Bell, M.A.L.: A deep learning based alternative to beamforming ultrasound images (2018)
15. Park, S., Karpiouk, A.B., Aglyamov, S.R., Emelianov, S.Y.: Adaptive beamforming for photoacoustic imaging. Opt. Lett. **33**(12), 1291–1293 (2008)
16. Treeby, B.E., Cox, B.T.: k-Wave: MATLAB toolbox for the simulation and reconstruction of photoacoustic wave fields. J. Biomed. Opt. **15**(2), 021314 (2010)
17. Yu, F., Koltun, V.: Multi-scale context aggregation by dilated convolutions. arXiv preprint arXiv:1511.07122 (2015)
18. Zhang, H.K., et al.: Prostate specific membrane antigen (PSMA)-targeted photoacoustic imaging of prostate cancer in vivo. J. Biophotonics **13**, e201800021 (2018)

A Training Tool for Ultrasound-Guided Central Line Insertion with Webcam-Based Position Tracking

Mark Asselin$^{(\boxtimes)}$, Tamas Ungi, Andras Lasso, and Gabor Fichtinger

Laboratory for Percutaneous Surgery,
Queen's University, Kingston, ON K7L 2N8, Canada
{mark.asselin, ungi, lasso, fichting}@queensu.ca

Abstract. PURPOSE: This paper describes an open-source ultrasound-guided central line insertion training system. Modern clinical guidelines are increasingly recommending ultrasound guidance for this procedure due to the decrease in morbidity it provides. However, there are no adequate low-cost systems for helping new clinicians train their inter-hand coordination for this demanding procedure. METHODS: This paper details a training platform which can be recreated with any standard ultrasound machine using inexpensive components. We describe the hardware, software, and calibration procedures with the intention that a reader can recreate this system themselves. RESULTS: The reproducibility and accuracy of the ultrasound calibration for this system was examined. We found that across the ultrasound image the calibration error was less than 2 mm. In a small feasibility study, two participants performed 5 needle insertions each with an average of slightly above 2 mm error. CONCLUSION: We conclude that the accuracy of the system is sufficient for clinician training.

Keywords: Open-source · Webcam tracking · Central line insertion
Medical training

1 Introduction

Central line insertion is the placement of a catheter usually through a major vein in the neck for administering medication and fluids directly into the heart. This common procedure is routinely performed to directly monitor venous pressure, to deliver large volumes of fluids, or to infuse solutions that would harm peripheral veins.

In many countries, the standard of care for central line insertion includes the use of ultrasound (US) guidance [1]. Ultrasound helps the operator find the optimal needle insertion location at the first insertion attempt, and helps prevent accidental puncture of the carotid artery. US is also used to visualize a patients' anatomy and provide guidance during the insertion of the needle. To insert a needle under US guidance, a clinician must simultaneously manipulate an ultrasound probe and the needle, one in each hand. Maintaining this coordination amidst the many steps of a venous cannulation is a daunting task for new clinicians. This problem is compounded by a lack of accessible practical training tools for medical students and clinician trainees to practice this coordination. In this paper we detail an inexpensive and portable system designed

© Springer Nature Switzerland AG 2018
D. Stoyanov et al. (Eds.): POCUS 2018/BIVPCS 2018/CuRIOUS 2018/CPM 2018,
LNCS 11042, pp. 12–20, 2018.
https://doi.org/10.1007/978-3-030-01045-4_2

to foster this skill in new clinicians by real time position tracking of the instruments for virtual reality visualization.

1.1 Standard Procedure for Central Line Insertion

To perform central line insertion, a clinician will first select a vein for catheterization. Typical sites include the internal jugular vein (in the neck), the femoral vein (in the thigh), or the subclavian vein (in the upper chest). In this paper we focus on internal jugular vein insertions, but the skills developed apply equally to using US guidance at any of the three sites [2].

Once the clinician has selected the insertion site, they will examine the patient's anatomy and attempt to discriminate between the vein and other nearby structures, including arteries, nerves and the surrounding tissues. This step is crucially important. Accidental cannulation of the artery is a serious complication in this procedure with the potential to cause significant morbidity or mortality [3]. Other serious complications include pneumothorax (collapsed lung), infection, air embolus, and losing the guide-wire into the vasculature. To help avoid these complications, many modern clinical guidelines suggest the use of ultrasound when performing central line insertion. US guidance is especially effective for helping to discern the artery from the vein. In a 900-patient randomized study, Karakitsos et al. compared the use of ultrasound against anatomical landmarks for central line insertion. They found a significant reduction in access time, as well as significant reductions in many of the common complications [4]. For these reasons, modern clinical standards are recommending the use of US guidance for this procedure.

There are two common techniques for the positioning of the ultrasound probe relative to the vein for the needle insertion. The first technique is called an "out of plane" insertion, where the imaging plane bisects the vein at a right angle. Out of plane insertion provides excellent visualization of the vein and the artery, helping to prevent accidental arterial cannulation. The two vessels can be distinguished by their relative positions within the anatomy. However, the drawback of the out of plane insertion method is that the operator must advance the needle and the probe iteratively, being very careful not to advance the needle ahead of the US imaging plane. If this were to happen, the operator would lose visualization of the advancing needle's path.

The second common technique for central line insertion is an "in plane" insertion where the US plane is parallel to the vessel. This technique has the advantage of continuous needle tip visualization, at the expense of making it more difficult to distinguish the artery from the vein. Hybrid techniques have been suggested where the clinician holds the probe at an oblique angle relative to the vein. This is intended to combine the advantages of the in plane and out of plane insertions [5]. In this paper we demonstrate our visualization with the out of plane approach, though it can be easily used for the in plane or oblique approaches by rotating the probe.

1.2 Training Challenges

One of the major challenges faced by new clinicians learning to use US guidance for needle insertion is the development of the requisite hand coordination. Clinicians must be able to simultaneously control the US probe in one hand, and the needle in the other. We have found in earlier studies that 3-dimensional visualization of the ultrasound image and the needle in real time is an effective training tool in learning coordination skills in ultrasound-guided needle placement [6]. This training setup requires position tracking of the ultrasound and the needle. Position tracking has additional advantages besides enabling 3-dimensional visualization as a training tool. Tracking can be used for the quantification of trainee skills for objective competency assessment [7], and for providing real time information to the trainee on the next procedure steps to perform in the early phases of training [8].

Although position tracking of the ultrasound and needle has many advantages during training of central line insertion, it is currently an expensive and complicated system. In this paper, we aim to show how a tracking system can be built for central line training using only open-source software and an inexpensive webcam for optical tracking. We evaluate the reproducibility and accuracy of the system and perform a small feasibility study.

2 Methods

2.1 Hardware

One major barrier in training new clinicians for US guided central line catheterization is the high cost for specialized, non-portable hardware. In creating this system we used only off the shelf components that are robust and relatively inexpensive to obtain. The design of every custom tool we used is open-sourced and the tools can be printed on any inexpensive 3D printer. Excluding the computer and the US machine, the total hardware cost for this system is ∼$200 US. The system can be built around any computer and any ultrasound machine; we endeavor to describe the system assembly in enough detail to allow it to be replicated easily. Additional instructions, source files, screenshots and information are available on the project's GitHub page[1].

In our experiments, we used a modern Lenovo laptop computer and a Telemed USB ultrasound with a L12 linear probe (Telemed Ltd., Lithuania). We have found this portable ultrasound machine to be incredibly suitable for US training applications. In addition to this, we used an Intel RealSense D415 depth camera (Intel, California, USA). We chose this camera in particular because it has fixed focus. We have found in the past that webcam autofocus can cause interruptions in tracking. Another advantage of this camera is its integrated depth sensor, capable of producing a point cloud of the scene in front of it. We envision several possible extensions to this system which would make use of this feature.

In addition to the components we purchased, we needed to design and manufacture several tools shown in Fig. 1. The STL models and source files for all these tools are open source, and accessible on the project's GitHub page and in the PLUS model

---

[1] Project Github page: https://github.com/SlicerIGT/OMTCentralLineTraining.

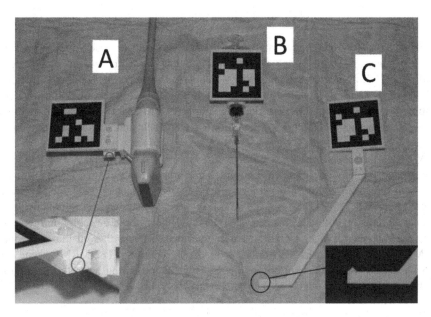

Fig. 1. Open source 3D printed tools with ArUco markers for tracking. A: ultrasound probe with marker bracket, embedded pivot calibration dimple is circled in red. B: tracked syringe mounted to steel needle. C: tracked stylus for US calibration, note the pointed tip. (Color figure online)

repository[2]. Each tool has a black and white marker to be used with the ArUco marker tracking toolkit [9]. The first tool (A) is a clip to connect an ArUco marker to the US probe. This clip also has a built-in dimple for performing pivot calibration. The middle tool (B) is a marker plane to rigidly fix an ArUco marker to the syringe. The hockey stick shaped tool (C) is a tracked stylus used to perform the calibration needed to visualize the US image in 3D space. To create these components, we used the Autodesk Fusion 360 (Autodesk, California, USA) CAD software to create the STL models. We then 3D printed these on an inexpensive 3D printer (Qidi Tech, Rui'an, China).

An important consideration when creating these tracked tools is the orientation of the marker with respect to the tracker. This is important to maintain good tracking accuracy. The goal is to ensure the plane of the ArUco marker is close to perpendicular to a ray drawn between the tracker and the center of the marker. This consideration must be balanced against ergonomic constraints and marker occlusion avoidance. We have found the use of 3D printing to be a useful tool in solving this problem because it enables the rapid creation of iterative prototypes. Typically it takes multiple prototypes to arrive at a satisfactory design.

---

[2] PLUS Toolkit open source model catalog, accessible at: http://perk-software.cs.queensu.ca/plus/doc/nightly/modelcatalog/.

2.2 System Design

To capture real-time US frames and tracking data we used the PLUS toolkit [10]. In order to track the tools using the Intel RealSense webcam, we used the OpticalMarkerTracking device built into PLUS [11]. This software device allows tracking to be performed using any RGB webcam, including the webcams built into modern laptops. It leverages the ArUco marker tracking toolkit to enable distortion correction of the camera image and pose computation of the black and white patterns shown above.

We built the visualization and training software on top of 3D Slicer, a widely used open-source application framework for medical image computing. Specifically, we leveraged the functionality in the image guided therapy extension built for 3D Slicer called SlicerIGT [12]. Using these two tools, this system was assembled without writing any custom software. Instead, we created a Slicer scene through configuration of Slicer widgets in Slicer's graphical user interface. Then we saved the scene into MRML file, an XML-based file format for medical computing. The MRML scene can then be loaded from Slicer on any computer (Fig. 2), providing an easy distribution mechanism for software developed in this manner.

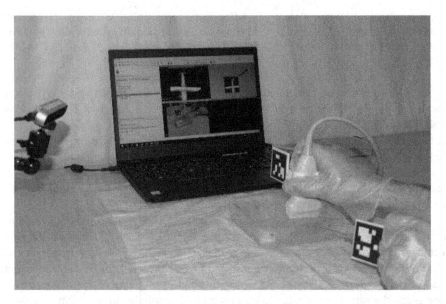

Fig. 2. The complete training system in use.

2.3 Calibration

One of the critical steps in building any tracked ultrasound system is to calibrate the US image with respect to the position sensor mounted on the US probe. This process is typically referred to as ultrasound calibration. To calibrate this training tool, we used a fiducial based registration procedure. The general idea of this method is to track the positions of the stylus and probe, using corresponding points in each frame of reference to determine the transformation between the two coordinate systems. This process begins by computing the tip of the stylus in its own coordinate system via pivot calibration. Then, a sampling of points distributed across the US image are collected along with their corresponding points in 3D space. We typically choose to use 6–10 such points in our calibrations. In Fig. 3, the selection of a sample point is shown. The position of the stylus tip is recorded in the US image (top left quadrant) and in 3D space (top right quadrant). The frame of video data from the webcam-based marker tracking is shown in the bottom left quadrant for reference. A more detailed description of this calibration process can be found in the SlicerIGT tracked ultrasound calibration tutorial[3].

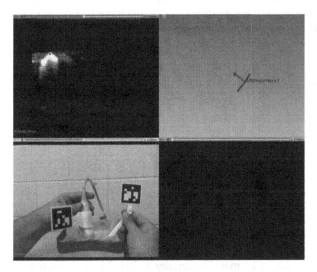

Fig. 3. Selection of points during US calibration. Top left: stylus tip position in US image coordinates. Top right: stylus tip position in 3D space. Bottom left: image of stylus & US probe from which tracking data was computed.

2.4   Calibration Verification

To verify the reproducibility of our US calibration, we performed a sequence of 5 calibrations. We then placed imaginary points in 5 regions of interest in the US frame - the center and each of the four corners. The center was selected because it is typically where the target for needle insertion will be, and the corners because any rotational error in the calibration will be most significant there. We transformed each of these points to physical space using all 5 of the US calibrations resulting in 5 clusters of 5 points each. For each cluster of 5, we took the center of mass as our best approximation to the true physical space position of the point. We then computed the average distance of the points in each cluster from the approximation of the true spatial position.

---

[3] SlicerIGT tracked ultrasound calibration tutorial: http://www.slicerigt.org/wp/user-tutorial/.

Lastly, we tested the system by having 2 users, one experienced with ultrasound and the other an intermediate operator, perform 5 needle insertions each. For each insertion, the operator targeted a 2 mm steel sphere implanted into a clear plastisol phantom. To assess their accuracy, we measured the maximum distance between the center of their needle tip and the closest side of the steel sphere. During the insertion the users were requested not to look directly at the phantom, relying only on the display of the training system.

3 Results

For each of the 5 calibration trials we recorded the root mean square (RMS) error of the pivot and fiducial registrations (Table 1). Note that these RMS errors are not a metric of accuracy, however they are a good measurement of the reproducibility of the system.

Table 1. RMS error from each pivot calibrations and corresponding fiducial registration.

Calibration #	Pivot RMS Error (mm)	FRE (RMS, mm)
1	0.41	1.31
2	0.55	1.92
3	0.58	1.47
4	0.46	1.78
5	0.53	1.41
Mean (STD)	0.51 (0.06)	1.58 (0.23)

Using each of the 5 US calibrations, we mapped 5 fiducials into their 3D positions using the image to probe transformation. The average distance of the 5 fiducials in each region from their center of mass is summarized in Table 2. Then using the best US calibration, two participants performed 5 needle localizations each on a simulated phantom using only the training system for guidance. The average distance from the simulated target for each participant is shown in Table 3.

Table 2. US calibration errors.

Region of Interest	Average Distance (mm)
Top Left	1.21
Top Right	1.64
Center	1.51
Bottom Left	1.49
Bottom Right	1.99

Table 3. Target localization errors.

Participant	Average distance from target mm (SD)
Intermediate	2.16 (1.10)
Experienced	2.32 (0.82)

4   Discussion

Overall, the errors in the calibration of the system fall within an acceptable target range for use in US guided needle insertion training.

Participants noted that an advantage of using the clear phantom is the immediate spatial feedback it provides post-localization. After each insertion participants could look at the phantom and quickly see where their needle was placed with respect to the target (Fig. 4). The authors feel that this may be an effective feedback for honing ability with this technique.

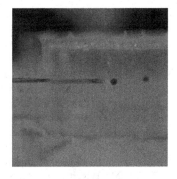

Fig. 4. Needle localization seen through clear phantom.

4.1   Limitations of Methods

The measurement of the needle to target sphere distance using calipers is subject to optical distortion in the clear phantom. To mitigate this, the phantom was designed with flat sides to minimize the lens effect. Ideally, we would have measured the needle – sphere distance using X-Ray or CT imaging, but these modalities were infeasible in the confines of this preliminary study.

4.2   Potential Improvements

Our lab currently develops a system called Central Line Tutor, which provides guidance to trainees learning the sequence of steps for performing US guided central line insertion. It would be a straightforward exercise to integrate these two platforms, providing a complete low-cost toolkit for central line insertion training.

5   Conclusion

We have demonstrated the feasibility of using a webcam-based system for training new clinicians hand coordination for ultrasound guided central line insertion. Our training platform focused on developing the requisite inter-hand coordination for performing the needle insertion portion of the procedure.

Acknowledgement. This work was funded, in part, by NIH/NIBIB and NIH/NIGMS (via grant 1R01EB021396-01A1 - Slicer + PLUS: Point-of-Care Ultrasound) and by CANARIE's Research Software Program. Gabor Fichtinger is supported as a Cancer Care Ontario Research Chair in Cancer Imaging. Mark Asselin is supported by an NSERC USRA.

References

1. Frykholm, P., et al.: Clinical guidelines on central venous catheterization. Acta Anaethesiol Scand. **58**, 508–524 (2014). https://doi.org/10.1111/aas.12295
2. Rigby, I., Howes, D., Lord, J., Walker, I.: Central Venous Access. Resuscitation Education Consortium/Kingston Resuscitation Institute
3. Gillman, L.M., Blaivas, M., Lord, J., Al-Kadi, A., Kirkpatrick, A.W.: Ultrasound confirmation of guidewire position may eliminate accidental arterial dilation during central venous cannulation. Scand. J. Trauma, Resusc. Emerg. Med. **18**, 39–42 (2010). https://doi.org/10.1186/1757-7241-18-39
4. Karakitsos, D., et al.: Real-time ultrasound guided catheterization of the internal jugular vein: a prospective comparison with the landmark technique in critical care patients. Crit. Care **10**(6), R162 (2006). https://doi.org/10.1186/cc5101
5. Phelan, M., Hagerty, D.: The oblique view: an alternative approach for ultrasound-guided central line placement. J. Emerg. Med. **37**(4), 403–408 (2008). https://doi.org/10.1016/j.jemermed.2008.02.061
6. Keri, Z., et al.: Training for ultrasound-guided lumbar puncture on abnormal spines using an augmented reality system. Can. J. Anesth. **62**(7), 777–784 (2015). https://doi.org/10.1007/s12630-015-0367-2
7. Clinkard, D., et al.: The development and validation of hand motion analysis to evaluate competency in central line catheterization. Acad. Emerg. Med. **22**(2), 212–218 (2015). https://doi.org/10.1111/acem.12590
8. Hisey, R., Ungi, T., Holden, M., Baum, Z., Keri, Z., Fichtinger, G.: Real-time workflow detection using webcam video for providing real-time feedback in central venous catheterization training. In: SPIE Medical Imaging 2018, 10–15 February, Houston, Texas, USA (2018)
9. Garrido-Jurado, S., Munoz-Salinas, R., Madrid-Cuevas, F.J., Marin-Jimenes, M.J.: Automatic generation and detection of highly reliable fiducial markers under occlusion. Pattern Recogn. **47**(6), 2280–2292 (2014). https://doi.org/10.1016/j.patcog.2014.01.005
10. Lasso, A., Heffter, T., Rankin, A., Pinter, C., Ungi, T., Fichtinger, G.: PLUS: open-source toolkit for ultrasound-guided intervention systems. IEEE Trans Biomed Eng. **61**(10), 2527–2537 (2014). https://doi.org/10.1109/tbme.2014.2322864
11. Asselin, M., Lasso, A., Ungi, T., Fichtinger, G.: Towards webcam-based tracking for interventional navigation. In: SPIE Medical Imaging 2018, 10–15 February, Houston, Texas, USA (2018)
12. Ungi, T., Lasso, A., Fichtinger, G.: Open-source platforms for navigated image-guided interventions. Med. Image Anal. **33**, 181–186 (2016)

GLUENet: Ultrasound Elastography Using Convolutional Neural Network

Md. Golam Kibria[1(✉)] and Hassan Rivaz[1,2(✉)]

[1] Concordia University, Montreal, QC, Canada
m_kibri@encs.concordia.ca, hrivaz@ece.concordia.ca
[2] PERFORM Centre, Montreal, QC, Canada

Abstract. Displacement estimation is a critical step in ultrasound elastography and failing to estimate displacement correctly can result in large errors in strain images. As conventional ultrasound elastography techniques suffer from decorrelation noise, they are prone to fail in estimating displacement between echo signals obtained during tissue deformations. This study proposes a novel elastography technique which addresses the decorrelation in estimating displacement field. We call our method GLUENet (GLobal Ultrasound Elastography Network) which uses deep Convolutional Neural Network (CNN) to get a coarse but robust time-delay estimation between two ultrasound images. This displacement is later used for formulating a nonlinear cost function which incorporates similarity of RF data intensity and prior information of estimated displacement [3]. By optimizing this cost function, we calculate the finer displacement exploiting all the information of all the samples of RF data simultaneously. The coarse displacement estimate generated by CNN is substantially more robust than the Dynamic Programming (DP) technique used in GLUE for finding the coarse displacement estimates. Our results validate that GLUENet outperforms GLUE in simulation, phantom and *in-vivo* experiments.

Keywords: Convolutional neural network · Ultrasound elastography
Time-delay estimation · TDE · Deep learning · Global elastography

1 Introduction

Ultrasound elastography can provide mechanical properties of tissue in real-time, and as such, has an important role in point-of-care ultrasound. Estimation of tissue deformation is very important in elastography, and further has numerous other applications such as thermal imaging [9] and echocardiography [1].

Over the last two decades, many techniques have been reported for estimating tissue deformation using ultrasound. The most common approach is window-based methods with cross-correlation matching techniques. Some reported these techniques in temporal domain [5, 10, 14] while others reported in spectral domain

© Springer Nature Switzerland AG 2018
D. Stoyanov et al. (Eds.): POCUS 2018/BIVPCS 2018/CuRIOUS 2018/CPM 2018,
LNCS 11042, pp. 21–28, 2018.
https://doi.org/10.1007/978-3-030-01045-4_3

[8,11]. Another notable approach for estimating tissue deformation is usage of dynamic programming with regularization and analytic minimization [3,12]. All these approaches may fail when severe decorrelation noise exists between ultrasound images.

Tissue deformation estimation in ultrasound images is an analogous to the optical flow estimation problem in computer vision. The structure and elastic property of tissue impose the fact that tissue deformation must contain some degree of continuity. Hence, tissue deformation estimation can be considered as a special case of optical flow estimation which is not bound by structural continuity. Apart from many state-of-the-art conventional approaches for optical flow estimation, very recently notable success has been reported at using deep learning network for end-to-end optical flow estimation. Deep learning networks enjoy the benefit of very fast calculation by trained (fine-tuned) weights of the network while having a trade-off of long-time computationally exhaustive training phase. Deep learning has been recently applied to estimation of elasticity from displacement data [4]. A promising recent network called FlowNet 2.0 [6] has achieved up to 140 fps at optical flow estimation. These facts indicate the potential for using deep learning for tissue deformation estimation.

This work takes advantage of the fast FlowNet 2.0 architecture to estimate an initial time delay estimation which is robust from decorrelation noise. This initial estimation is then fine-tuned by optimizing a global cost function [3]. We call our method GLUENet (GLobal Ultrasound Elastography Network) and show that it has many advantages over conventional methods. The most important one would be the robustness of the method to severe decorrelation noise between ultrasound images.

2   Methods

The proposed method calculates the time delay between two radio-frequency (RF) ultrasound scans which are correlated by a displacement field in two phases combining fast and robust convolutional neural network with the more accurate global optimization based coarse to fine displacement estimation. This combination is possible due to the fact that the global optimization-based method depends on coarse but robust displacement estimation which CNN can provide readily and more robustly than any other state-of-the-art elastography method.

Optical flow estimation in computer vision and tissue displacement estimation in ultrasound elastography share common challenges. Therefore, optical flow estimation techniques can be used for tissue displacement estimation for ultrasound elastography. The latest CNN that can estimate optical flow with competitive accuracy with the state-of-the-art conventional methods is called FlowNet 2.0 [6]. This network is an improved version of its predecessor FlowNet [2], wherein Dosovitskiy et al. trained two basic networks namely FlowNetS and FlowNetC for optical flow prediction. FlowNetC is a customized network for optical flow estimation whereas FlowNetS is rather a generic network. The details of these networks can be found in [2]. These networks were further improved for more accuracy in [6] which is known as FlowNet 2.0.

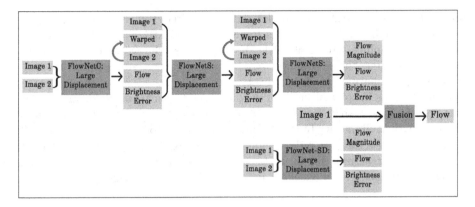

Fig. 1. Full schematic of FlowNet 2.0 architecture: The initial network input is Image 1 and Image 2. The input of the subsequent networks includes the image pairs, previously estimated flow, Image 2 warped with the flow, and residual of Image 1 and warped image (Brightness error). Input data is concatenated (indicated by braces).

Figure 1 illustrates the complete schematic of FlowNet 2.0 architecture. It can be considered as the stacked version of a combination of FlowNetC and FlowNetS architectures which help the network to calculate large displacement optical flow. For dealing with the small displacements, small strides were introduced in the beginning of the FlowNetS architecture. In addition to that, convolution layers were introduced between upconvolutions for smoothing. Finally, the final flow is estimated using a fusion network. The details can be found in [6].

The displacement estimation from FlowNet 2.0 is robust but needs more refinement in order to produce strain images of high quality. Global Time-Delay Estimation (GLUE) [3] is an accurate displacement estimation method provided that an initial coarse displacement estimation is available. If the initial displacement estimation contains large errors, then GLUE may fail to produce accurate fine displacement estimation. GLUE refines the initial displacement estimation by optimizing a cost function incorporating both amplitude similarity and displacement continuity. It is noteworthy that the cost function is formulated for the entire image unlike its motivational previous work [12] where only a single RF line is optimized. The details of the cost function and its optimization can be found in [3]. After displacement refinement, strain image is obtained by using least square or a Kalman filter [12].

3   Results

GLUENet is evaluated using simulation and experimental phantom, and *in-vivo* patient data. The simulation phantom contains a soft inclusion in the middle and the corresponding displacement is calculated using Finite Element Method (FEM) by ABAQUS Software (Providence, RI). For ultrasound simulation, the Field II software package [7] is used. A CIRS breast phantom (Norfolk, VA) is used as the experimental phantom. RF data is acquired using an Antares Siemens system (Issaquah, WA) at the center frequency of 6.67 MHz with a VF10-5 linear array at a sampling rate of 40 MHz. For clinical study, we used *in-vivo* data of three patients. These patients were undergoing open surgical RF thermal ablation for primary or secondary liver cancer. The *in-vivo* data were collected at John Hopkins Hospital. Details of the data acquisition are available in [12]. For comparison of the robustness of our method, we use mathematical metrics such as Mean Structural Similarity Index (MSSIM) [13], Signal to Noise Ratio (SNR) and Contrast to Noise Ratio (CNR). Among them, MSSIM incorporates luminance, contrast, and structural similarity between ground truth and estimated strain images which makes it an excellent indicator of perceived image quality.

3.1   Simulation Results

Field II RF data with strains ranging from 0.5% to 7% are simulated, and uniformly distributed random noise with PSNR of 12.7 dB is added to the RF data. The additional noise is for illustrating the robustness of the method to decorrelation noise given that simulation does not model out-of-plane motion of the probe, complex biological motion, and electronic noise. Figure 2(a) shows ground truth axial strain and (b–c) shows axial strains generated by GLUE and GLUENet respectively at 2% applied strain. Figure 2(d–f) illustrates the comparable performance of GLUENet against GLUE [3] in terms of MSSIM, SNR and CNR respectively.

3.2   Experimental Phantom Results

Figure 3(a–b) shows axial strains of the CIRS phantom generated by GLUE and GLUENet respectively. The large blue and red windows in Fig. 3(a–b) are used as target and background windows for calculating SNR and CNR (Table 1). The small windows are moved to create a total combination of 120 window pairs (6 as target and 20 as background) for calculating CNR values. The histogram of these CNR values is plotted in Fig. 3(c) to provide a more comprehensive view which shows that GLUENet has a high frequency at high CNR values while GLUE is highly frequent at lower values. We test both methods on 62 pre- and post- compression RF signal pairs chosen from 20 RF signals of CIRS phantom for a measure of consistency. The best among the estimated strain images is visually marked to compare with other strain images using Normalized Cross Correlation (NCC). A threshold at 0.6 is used to determine failure rate of the methods (Table 1). GLUENet shows very low failure rate (19.3548%) compared to GLUE (58.0645%) which indicates greater consistency of GLUENet.

3.3   Clinical Results

Figure 4 shows axial strains of patient 1–3 from GLUE and GLUENet and histogram of CNR values. Similar to experimental phantom data, small target and

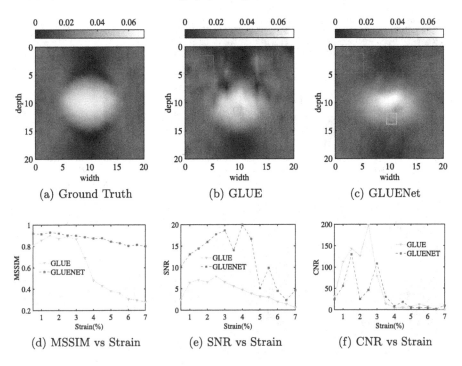

(a) Ground Truth   (b) GLUE   (c) GLUENet

(d) MSSIM vs Strain   (e) SNR vs Strain   (f) CNR vs Strain

Fig. 2. First row shows axial strain images of simulation phantom with added random noise (PSNR: 12.7 dB); (a) Ground truth, (b) GLUE and (c) GLUENet. Second row shows the performance metrics graph with respect to various range of applied strain; (d) MSSIM vs Strain, (e) SNR vs Strain and (f) CNR vs Strain.

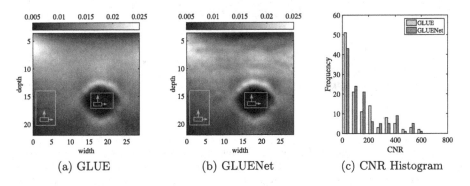

(a) GLUE   (b) GLUENet   (c) CNR Histogram

Fig. 3. Axial strain images of experimental phantom data generated by (a) GLUE and (b) GLUENet, and (c) histogram of CNR values of GLUE and GLUENet. (Color figure online)

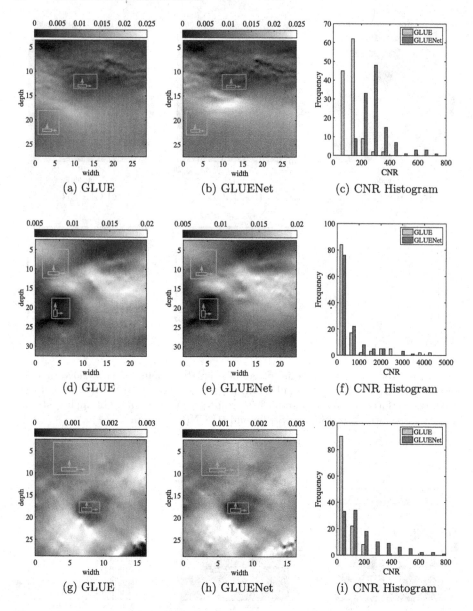

Fig. 4. Axial strain images of patients and histogram of CNR values: The three rows correspond to patients 1–3 respectively. First and second columns depict axial strain images from GLUE and GLUENet respectively. Third column shows histogram of CNR values of GLUE and GLUENet. (Color figure online)

Table 1. SNR and CNR of the strain images, and failure rate of GLUE and GLUENet for experimental phantom data and *in-vivo* data of patients 1–3.

	GLUE			GLUENet		
	SNR	CNR	Failure rate (%)	SNR	CNR	Failure rate (%)
Phantom	39.0363	12.6588	58.0645	43.4363	15.5291	19.3548
Patient 1	53.9914	22.1641	34.6939	54.7700	27.9264	04.8469
Patient 2	47.5051	22.7523	68.3673	55.9494	25.4911	14.5408
Patient 3	31.2440	07.7831	77.0408	28.6152	19.6954	60.7143

background windows are moved to create a total combination of 120 window pairs for calculating CNR values. Their histogram shows that GLUENet has a high frequency at high CNR values while GLUE is more frequent at low values. Table 1 shows the SNR and CNR values for all patients which is calculated by using the large blue and red windows as target and background. We calculate failure rate of GLUE and GLUENet from 392 pre- and post- compression RF echo frame pairs chosen from 60 RF echo frames of all three patients. The best axial strain is marked visually to compare with other strains using NCC. A threshold of 0.6 is used to determine the failure rate of the methods shown in Table 1. The failure rate of GLUENet is very low compared to GLUE for all patient data thus proving the robustness of GLUENet to decorrelation noise in clinical data.

The failure rates of GLUE in Table 1 are generally high because no parameter tuning is performed for the hyperparameters. Another reason for high failure rates is that we select pairs of frames that are temporally far from each other to test the robustness at extreme levels. This substantially increases non-axial motion of the probe and complex biological motions, which leads to severe decorrelation in the RF signal. In real-life, the failure rate of these methods can be improved by selecting pairs of RF data that are not temporally far from each other.

4   Conclusions

In this paper, we introduced a novel technique to calculate tissue displacement from ultrasound images using CNN. This is, to the best of our knowledge, the first use of CNN for estimation of displacement in ultrasound elastography. The displacement estimation obtained from CNN was further refined using GLUE [3], and therefore, we referred to our method as GLUENet. We showed that GLUENet is robust to decorrelation noise in simulation, experiments and *in-vivo* data, which makes it a good candidate for clinical use. In addition, the high robustness to noise allows elastography to be performed by less experienced sonographers as a point-of-care imaging tool.

Acknowledgement. This research has been supported in part by NSERC Discovery Grant (RGPIN-2015-04136). We would like to thank Microsoft Azure Research for a cloud computing grant and NVIDIA for GPU donation. The ultrasound data was collected at Johns Hopkins Hospital. The principal investigators were Drs. E. Boctor, M. Choti, and G. Hager. We thank them for sharing the data with us.

References

1. Amundsen, B.H., et al.: Noninvasive myocardial strain measurement by speckle tracking echocardiography: validation against sonomicrometry and tagged magnetic resonance imaging. J. Am. Coll. Cardiol. **47**(4), 789–793 (2006)
2. Dosovitskiy, A., et al.: FlowNet: learning optical flow with convolutional networks. In: Proceedings of the IEEE International Conference on Computer Vision, pp. 2758–2766 (2015)
3. Hashemi, H.S., Rivaz, H.: Global time-delay estimation in ultrasound elastography. IEEE Trans. Ultrason. Ferroelectr. Freq. Control **64**(10), 1625–1636 (2017)
4. Hoerig, C., Ghaboussi, J., Insana, M.F.: An information-based machine learning approach to elasticity imaging. Biomech. Model Mechanobiol. **16**(3), 805–822 (2017)
5. Hussain, M.A., Anas, E.M.A., Alam, S.K., Lee, S.Y., Hasan, M.K.: Direct and gradient-based average strain estimation by using weighted nearest neighbor cross-correlation peaks. IEEE TUFFC **59**(8), 1713–1728 (2012)
6. Ilg, E., Mayer, N., Saikia, T., Keuper, M., Dosovitskiy, A., Brox, T.: FlowNet 2.0: evolution of optical flow estimation with deep networks. In: IEEE Conference on Computer Vision and Pattern Recognition (CVPR), vol. 2 (2017)
7. Jensen, J.A.: FIELD: a program for simulating ultrasound systems. Med. Biol. Eng. Comput. **34**(suppl. 1, pt. 1), 351–353 (1996)
8. Kibria, M.G., Hasan, M.K.: A class of kernel based real-time elastography algorithms. Ultrasonics **61**, 88–102 (2015)
9. Kim, Y., Audigier, C., Ziegle, J., Friebe, M., Boctor, E.M.: Ultrasound thermal monitoring with an external ultrasound source for customized bipolar RF ablation shapes. IJCARS **13**(6), 815–826 (2018)
10. Ophir, J., et al.: Elastography: imaging the elastic properties of soft tissues with ultrasound. J. Med. Ultra. **29**(4), 155–171 (2002)
11. Pesavento, A., Perrey, C., Krueger, M., Ermert, H.: A time-efficient and accurate strain estimation concept for ultrasonic elastography using iterative phase zero estimation. IEEE TUFFC **46**(5), 1057–1067 (1999)
12. Rivaz, H., Boctor, E.M., Choti, M.A., Hager, G.D.: Real-time regularized ultrasound elastography. IEEE Trans. Med. Imaging **30**(4), 928–945 (2011)
13. Wang, Z., Bovik, A.C., Sheikh, H.R., Simoncelli, E.P.: Image quality assessment: from error visibility to structural similarity. IEEE TIP **13**(4), 600–612 (2004)
14. Zahiri-Azar, R., Salcudean, S.E.: Motion estimation in ultrasound images using time domain cross correlation. IEEE TMB **53**(10), 1990–2000 (2006)

CUST: CNN for Ultrasound Thermal Image Reconstruction Using Sparse Time-of-Flight Information

Younsu Kim[1], Chloé Audigier[1], Emran M. A. Anas[1], Jens Ziegle[2], Michael Friebe[2], and Emad M. Boctor[1(✉)]

[1] Johns Hopkins University, Baltimore, MD, USA
eboctor1@jhmi.edu
[2] Otto-von-Guericke University, Magdeburg, Germany

Abstract. Thermotherapy is a clinical procedure to induce a desired biological tissue response through temperature changes. To precisely operate the procedure, temperature monitoring during the treatment is essential. Ultrasound propagation velocity in biological tissue changes as temperature increases. An external ultrasound element was integrated with a bipolar radiofrequency (RF) ablation probe to collect time-of-flight information carried by ultrasound waves going through the ablated tissues. Recovering temperature at the pixel level from the limited information acquired from this minimal setup is an ill-posed problem. Therefore, we propose a learning approach using a designed convolutional neural network. Training and testing were performed with temperature images generated with a computational bioheat model simulating a RF ablation. The reconstructed thermal images were compared with results from another sound velocity reconstruction method. The proposed method showed better stability and accuracy for different ultrasound element locations. *Ex-vivo* experiments were also performed on porcine liver to evaluate the proposed temperature reconstruction method.

Keywords: Ultrasound thermal monitoring
Temperature image reconstruction · Bipolar ablation · Hyperthermia
Thermotherapy · CNN · Ultrasound

1 Introduction

Thermotherapy is a clinical procedure that uses thermal energy to induce a desired biological tissue response. Mild and localized hyperthermia can be used in combination with chemotherapy or drug delivery to improve the therapy response [1,2]. Thermal ablation can be achieved by applying sufficient thermal energy to reach a complete destruction of various kinds of cancer cells. However, the main challenge is to cover completely the target region while preserving

© Springer Nature Switzerland AG 2018
D. Stoyanov et al. (Eds.): POCUS 2018/BIVPCS 2018/CuRIOUS 2018/CPM 2018,
LNCS 11042, pp. 29–37, 2018.
https://doi.org/10.1007/978-3-030-01045-4_4

the surrounding healthy tissues. Monitoring the temperature across this region is necessary to control the delivered thermal energy and operating duration to precisely and successfully operate the procedure [3].

A widely accepted approach to measure temperature is the use of invasive thermometers [4]. However, it allows temperature monitoring only at a few spatial locations. Magnetic resonance imaging (MRI) is the current clinical standard to monitor the spatial temperature distribution [5]. In addition to the high cost of MRI, it requires the therapy instruments to be MR-compatible. Furthermore, MRI is not suitable for patients with pacemaker, neurostimulator or metal implants. An alternative is to use portable and affordable ultrasound (US) techniques, and a significant number of related works have been reported [6]. These approaches exploit the temperature dependent ultrasound properties such as sound velocity and attenuation to estimate the temperature. Sound velocity or attenuation images can be generated using ultrasound tomography techniques, which typically require extensive data acquisition from multiple angles. Ultrasound tomographic images can also be reconstructed using time-of-flight (TOF) information from limited angles using an isothermal model [7]. To overcome the sparsity of the data, machine learning is a promising alternative [8].

In this work, we propose a deep learning approach for tomographic reconstruction of sound velocity images. We collected TOFs using a clinical ultrasound transducer and by integrating an active ultrasound element on a bipolar radiofrequency (RF) ablation probe. The number of acquired TOFs is limited by the number of elements in the ultrasound transducer, usually insufficient to solve for the sound velocity in the heated region. Therefore, we implemented a convolutional neural network (CNN) to reconstruct temperature images using this limited information. For the training of the network, thermal images are generated with a computational bioheat model of RF ablation, and then converted to sound velocity images to obtain simulated TOF datasets. We performed simulation and *ex-vivo* experiments to evaluate the proposed method.

2   Methods

2.1   Thermal Ablation Procedure and Monitoring Setup

The thermal ablation procedure is performed with bipolar RF needles to generate various ablation patterns [9] and an active ultrasound element is used for temperature monitoring as shown in Fig. 1(a). As the element can be integrated with the ablation probe, it does not increase the overall invasiveness of the procedure. Two different ablation patterns were considered: horizontal and diagonal as illustrated in Fig. 1(b). We created the horizontal pattern by activating the two electrodes at the tips of the RF probes, and the diagonal pattern by activating crossing electrodes. During the procedure, the external ultrasound element transmits ultrasound pulses. TOF data are collected with an ultrasound transducer to detect the change in sound velocity. Therefore, the monitored region is the triangular area created between the ultrasound transducer and the element. It belongs to the monitoring image plane between the two RF probes showed

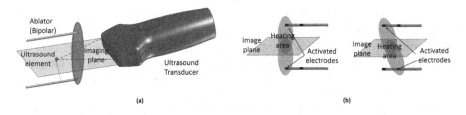

Fig. 1. (a) The ultrasound thermal monitoring setup. (b) Left: Horizontal ablation pattern. Right: Diagonal ablation pattern.

in Fig. 1. In this plane, the horizontal pattern showed a round-shaped temperature distribution, while the diagonal pattern showed an ellipsoid one.

2.2   Thermal Image Reconstruction Using Neural Network

Training Set Generation: A RFA computational model is used to simulate the temperature evolution in a 3D domain with various tissue parameters to provide temperature images for training. A reaction-diffusion equation (Eq. 1) following the Pennes bioheat model [10] is used:

$$\rho_t c_t \frac{\partial T}{\partial t} = Q + \nabla \cdot (d_t \nabla T) + R(T_{b0} - T) \tag{1}$$

where ρ_t, c_t, d_t are the density, heat capacity, and conductivity of the tissue. T_{b0}, R, Q, the blood temperature, reaction term, and source term modeling the heat from the ablation device. The implementation is based on the Lattice Boltzmann Method and inhomogeneous tissue structures can be considered [11]. To simulate RF ablation with bipolar probes, and thus various ablation lesion shapes, we assume the two RF electrodes as independent heating sources. Their temperatures are imposed as Dirichlet boundary conditions [11]. For each ablation pattern, we simulated a procedure of 8 min of heating followed by 2 min of cooling, which corresponds to 600 temperature images having a temporal resolution of 1 s. We wanted to mimic the *ex-vivo* experiment setup, therefore porcine tissue parameters were used, even though a shorter cooling period was achieved due to a data storage limitation in the current experimental setup [11]. For the horizontal pattern, the temperature range was between 22.0 °C and 37.8 °C, and for the diagonal pattern, between 23.0 °C and 35.9 °C.

Different ultrasound element locations can also be considered. We defined a 2D image coordinate system as (Axial, Lateral) axis in millimeter scale. The image plane was divided in 60 by 60 pixels. A 6 cm linear 128 element ultrasound probe was placed between (0, 0) and (0, 60), and the ultrasound element was located within the image plane. The network training set is made of those images as well as the corresponding simulated TOF information.

In order to simulate the acquisition of TOF dataset, we converted the temperature images into sound velocity images as the sound velocity within the tissue changes with temperature. Since the major component of biological tissue is water, the relationship between sound velocity and temperature for biological tissue has a trend similar to the water one [12]. In this paper, we used a converting equation acquired from a tissue-mimicking phantom with a sound velocity offset compensation [13] to simulate TOF information affected by a change in temperature and therefore in sound velocity even though a tissue-specific relationship could be used if the tissue type is known.

We simulated 49 different ultrasound element locations around the location used in the *ex-vivo* experiment, with the heating center kept fixed. For the horizontal pattern, we moved the element location from (36, 40.5) to (42, 46.5) by a 1 mm step in both lateral and axial directions. For the diagonal pattern, element locations between (43.5, 51) and (49.5, 57) were considered. For each of the 49 locations, data were split randomly with a 6:1 ratio between training and testing sets. Therefore, for each ablation pattern, the total number of samples was 29,400, split into 4,200 testing and 25,200 training sets. This large dataset may ensure an effective training of the network parameters without over-fitting.

Image Reconstruction Network: Figure 2 shows the temperature image reconstruction neural network, which consists of two fully connected layers wrapping series of CNN. The convolutional network is symmetrically designed, consisting of convolution and trans-convolution layers. After the convolution operation, each CNN layer includes a ReLU followed by a batch normalization operation.

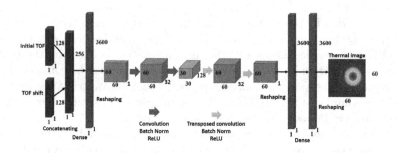

Fig. 2. Temperature image reconstruction network.

We concatenated the 128-length initial TOF vector with any TOF vector during the procedure into a 256-length input vector. The initial TOF is always used since it provides the element location and allows to access the TOF differences during the ablation procedure, valuable information for temperature reconstruction. As we reconstructed 3600 pixel temperature images with a 256-length input vector, we expanded the parameters at the beginning of the network.

Training Results: For each ablation pattern, we performed 1000 epochs using the Pytorch library [14]. Adam optimizer and mean squared error loss function were used. We compared the results to those obtained from another reconstruction method (CSRM) [13] in Table 1 at the 49 different ultrasound element locations. In this case, the ground truths are the simulated temperature

Table 1. Comparison of the CNN approach with a sound velocity reconstruction method using RFA modeling (CSRM) for the 49 different ultrasound element locations. The error is the difference of temperature in the imaging plane between the reconstructed image and the simulated image (ground truth).

Method	CSRM		CNN	
Pattern	Horizontal	Diagonal	Horizontal	Diagonal
Maximum errors (°C)	1.118 ± 2.701	0.788 ± 1.904	0.174 ± 0.198	0.064 ± 0.010
Mean errors (°C)	0.107 ± 0.243	0.070 ± 0.144	0.019 ± 0.018	0.011 ± 0.017

images. The CRSM method used an optimization approach with additional constraints brought by a computational RFA modeling. The CNN reconstruction method had 0.94 °C and 0.72 °C less maximum temperature error in the imaging plane than CSRM for the horizontal and diagonal pattern respectively. We also observed that the standard deviation decreased with the CNN approach. With the CSRM method, the reconstruction accuracy is highly affected by the ultrasound element location. Indeed, for certain locations, the ultrasound propagation paths may not intersect with the heating center. Among the 49 different element locations considered, the maximum error in the sound velocity reconstruction exceeds 5 m/s with CSRM at 7 and 2 locations for the horizontal and diagonal pattern respectively. The CNN reconstruction method showed less temperature error at those locations since it could estimate the temperature at the heating center more precisely using information learned from other temperature distributions.

We also tested with a fully connected network by replacing the middle structure with four dense networks which were the same as the last dense network in Fig. 2. The regression accuracy was similar to the CNN network with more parameters. To minimize over-fitting, we chose the hyper-parameters with the minimal number of layers maintaining the regression accuracy. The initial learning rate was 10^{-3}, and we re-trained with a smaller learning rate of 10^{-5}. We also tested our network without the last dense layers, the regression accuracy was inferior to the original network.

3   *Ex-vivo* Liver Ablation with Ultrasound Monitoring

3.1   Experiment Setup

Two *ex-vivo* porcine liver experiments were performed to test the performance of the trained model. Liver tissues were placed at room temperature for 12 h before performing the ablation. We used the setup illustrated in Fig. 1(a). Bipolar ablation probes were inserted 2-cm apart and in parallel by using a holder to perform horizontal and diagonal ablation patterns. The ablation power was provided by a RF generator (Radionics Inc., USA). The ultrasound element was placed within the porcine liver tissue. We adjusted its location to the ultrasound transducer

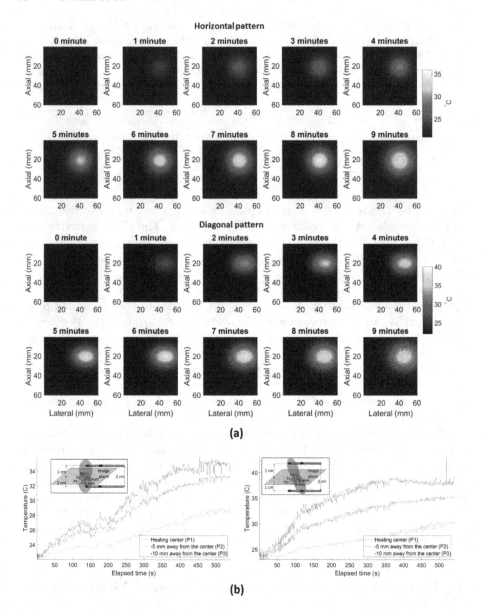

Fig. 3. Results of the *ex-vivo* experiments on porcine livers. (a) Temperature reconstruction for the horizontal and diagonal ablation patterns. (b) Temperature evolution over time at three different positions in the imaging plane. (Left): Horizontal ablation pattern. (Right): Diagonal ablation pattern.

by finding the maximum signal strength within the imaging plane. We used a 10 MHz linear transducer L14-5W/60 (Ultrasonix Corp., Canada) with a 5–14 MHz bandwidth and a SonixDAQ (Ultrasonix Corp., Canada) with a sampling frequency of 40 MHz. The ultrasound data was collected with a pitch-and-catch mode. The ultrasound element transmitted a pulse while the ultrasound transducer and DAQ received the signal simultaneously. The transmission and collection were synchronized by an external function generator at 1 Hz. We performed 8 min of ablation, after what the ablation probes remained in the tissue for an extra 1 min without RF power.

3.2   Temperature Image Reconstruction

TOF was detected by finding the first peak from the ultrasound channel data. The received signal had a center frequency of 3.7 MHz with a bandwidth of 2.5–5.6 MHz. During the two ablations, we collected 540 TOF dataset for 9 min. The element was localized at (39.0, 43.6) and (46.6, 54.2) in the horizontal and diagonal pattern experiments. We reconstructed temperature images using the model trained with the simulation datasets and we observed a convincing temperature trend over time. The temperature evolutions at three different points: heating center, -5 and -10 mm away from the center along the axial direction are shown in Fig. 3. The maximum TOF shift was 300 ns for the horizontal, and 475 ns for the diagonal pattern. In the horizontal pattern experiment, at around 180 and 230 s, the TOF increased for few samples compared to previous frames which was unexpected. This induced a temperature decrease at those time points. Nonetheless, we observed an overall temperature increase trend.

4   Discussion and Conclusion

As we use the relative changes in TOF to monitor the temperature during a thermal ablation, the complication of calculating the absolute sound velocity of different tissues is decreased. However, the variety of sound velocity changes against temperature in different tissue types may cause errors in the reconstructed temperature results. To overcome this problem, a calibration method for different tissue types can be used [13], and dataset from diverse tissue types should also be used to train the network. In this paper, the ablation power was limited due to the ongoing development of the bipolar ablation device, which limited the temperature range. But this method can be applied to ablation where higher temperatures are reached. Moreover, the *ex-vivo* experiment results could not be validated with other thermometry methods. MR-thermometry for example, was not an option since the ablation system is not MR-compatible. Thermocouples could block the ultrasound propagation paths, and only provide temperature information at few points. Therefore, we validated the method with simulation data, and observed an increasing temperature trend in *ex-vivo* experiments. Patient motion can affect the reconstruction accuracy, which is the main challenge for many ultrasound thermometry approaches. With our method, patient motion will change the location of the ultrasound element relative to the ultrasound transducer, which can be detected by a sudden change in TOF. The CNN model is trained with various ultrasound element locations, and the system could be further improved in the future to continue reconstructing temperature images using prior temperature information in the occurrence of patient motion.

Ultrasound is a preferable imaging modality due to its accessibility, cost-effectiveness, and non-ionizing nature. We have introduced a temperature monitoring method using an external ultrasound element and CNN. We have trained the model with simulation data, and applied it to *ex-vivo* experiments. One of the advantages of the proposed method is the fact that we can generate unlimited simulation datasets for the training. This method will be further extended for tomographic applications using sparse datasets.

Acknowledgments. This work was supported by the National Institute of Health (R01EB021396) and the National Science Foundation (1653322).

References

1. Landon, C.D., Park, J.Y., Needham, D., Dewhirst, M.W.: Nanoscale drug delivery and hyperthermia: the materials design and preclinical and clinical testing of low temperature-sensitive liposomes used in combination with mild hyperthermia in the treatment of local cancer. Open Nanomed. J. **3**, 38–64 (2011)
2. Issels, R.D.: Neo-adjuvant chemotherapy alone or with regional hyperthermia for localised high-risk soft-tissue sarcoma: a randomised phase 3 multicentre study. Lancet Oncol. **11**(6), 561–570 (2010)
3. Dinerman, J.L., Berger, R., Calkins, H.: Temperature monitoring during radiofrequency ablation. J. Cardiovasc. Electrophysiol. **7**(2), 163–173 (1996)
4. Saccomandi, P., Schena, E., Silvestri, S.: Techniques for temperature monitoring during laser-induced thermotherapy: an overview. Int. J. Hyperth. **29**(7), 609–619 (2013)
5. Poorter, J.D., Wagter, C.D., Deene, Y.D., Thomsen, C., Ståhlberg, F., Achten, E.: Noninvasive MRI thermometry with the proton resonance frequency (PRF) method: in vivo results in human muscle. Magn. Res. Med. **33**(1), 74–81 (1995)
6. Lewis, M.A., Staruch, R.M., Chopra, R.: Thermometry and ablation monitoring with ultrasound. Int. J. Hyperth. **31**(2), 163–181 (2015)
7. Norton, S.J., Testardi, L.R., Wadley, H.N.G.: Reconstructing internal temperature distributions from ultrasonic time-of-flight tomography and dimensional resonance measurements. In: 1983 Ultrasonics Symposium, pp. 850–855, October 1983
8. Wang, G.: A perspective on deep imaging. IEEE Access **4**, 8914–8924 (2016)
9. Ziegle, J., Audigier, C., Krug, J., Ali, G., Kim, Y., Boctor, E.M., Friebe, M.: RF-ablation pattern shaping employing switching channels of dual bipolar needle electrodes: ex vivo results. IJCARS, **13**, 1–12 (2018)
10. Pennes, H.H.: Analysis of tissue and arterial blood temperatures in the resting human forearm. J. Appl. Physiol. **85**(1), 5–34 (1998)
11. Audigier, C.: Efficient Lattice Boltzmann solver for patient-specific radiofrequency ablation of hepatic tumors. IEEE TMI **34**(7), 1576–1589 (2015)
12. Martnez-Valdez, R., Contreras, M., Vera, A., Leija, L.: Sound speed measurement of chicken liver from 22C to 60C. Phys. Procedia **70**, 1260–1263 (2015)

13. Kim, Y., Audigier, C., Ziegle, J., Friebe, M., Boctor, E.M.: Ultrasound thermal monitoring with an external ultrasound source for customized bipolar RF ablation shapes. IJCARS, **13**, 815–826 (2018)
14. Paszke, A., et al.: Automatic differentiation in pytorch (2017)

Quality Assessment of Fetal Head Ultrasound Images Based on Faster R-CNN

Zehui Lin[1,2,3], Minh Hung Le[1,2,3], Dong Ni[1,2,3], Siping Chen[1,2,3], Shengli Li[4], Tianfu Wang[1,2,3(✉)], and Baiying Lei[1,2,3(✉)]

[1] School of Biomedical Engineering, Shenzhen University, Shenzhen, China
{tfwang, leiby}@szu.edu.cn
[2] National-Regional Key Technology Engineering Laboratory for Medical Ultrasound, Shenzhen, China
[3] Guangdong Key Laboratory for Biomedical Measurements and Ultrasound Imaging, Shenzhen, China
[4] Department of Ultrasound, Affiliated Shenzhen Maternal and Child Healthcare, Hospital of Nanfang Medical University, Shenzhen, People's Republic of China

Abstract. Clinically, the transthalamic plane of the fetal head is manually examined by sonographers to identify whether it is a standard plane. This examination routine is subjective, time-consuming and requires comprehensive understanding of fetal anatomy. An automatic and effective computer aided diagnosis method to determine the standard plane in ultrasound images is highly desirable. This study presents a novel method for the quality assessment of fetal head in ultrasound images based on Faster Region-based Convolutional Neural Networks (Faster R-CNN). Faster R-CNN is able to learn and extract features from the training data. During the training, Fast R-CNN and Region Proposal Network (RPN) share the same feature layer through joint training and alternate optimization. The RPN generates more accurate region proposals, which are used as the inputs for the Fast R-CNN module to perform target detection. The network then outputs the detected categories and scores. Finally, the quality of the transthalamic plane is determined via the scores obtained from the numbers of detected anatomical structures. These scores detect the standard plane as well. Experimental results demonstrated that our method could accurately locate five specific anatomical structures of the transthalamic plane with an average accuracy of 80.18%, which takes only an approximately 0.27 s running time per image.

Keywords: Fetal head · Quality assessment · Ultrasound images
Faster R-CNN · Anatomical structure detection

1 Introduction

Ultrasound image has been preferred as an imaging modality for prenatal screening due to its noninvasive, real-time tracking, and low-cost. In prenatal diagnosis, it is important to obtain standard planes (e.g., the transthalamic plane) for prenatal ultrasound diagnosis. With the standard plane, doctors can measure the fetal physiological parameters to assess the growth and development of the fetus. Moreover, the weight of the fetus also can be obtained by measuring the parameters of biparietal diameter and

D. Stoyanov et al. (Eds.): POCUS 2018/BIVPCS 2018/CuRIOUS 2018/CPM 2018,
LNCS 11042, pp. 38–46, 2018.
https://doi.org/10.1007/978-3-030-01045-4_5

head circumference. This clinical practice is challenging for novices since it requires high-level clinical expertise and comprehensive understanding of fetal anatomy. Normally, ultrasound images scanned by novices are evaluated by experienced ultrasound doctors in the clinical practice, which is time-consuming and unappealing. To assist junior doctors by tracking the quality of the scanned image, automatic computer aided diagnosis for the quality assessment of ultrasound image is highly demanded. Accordingly, "intelligent ultrasound" [1] has become an inevitable trend due to the rapid development of image processing techniques. Powered by the machine learning and deep learning techniques, many dedicated research works have been proposed for this interesting topic, which mainly focus on the quality assessment of fetal ultrasound images to locate and identify the specific anatomical structures. For instance, Li *et al.* [2] combined Random Forests and medicine prior knowledge to detect the region of interest (ROI) of the fetal head circumference. Vaanathi *et al.* [3] utilized FCN architecture to detect the fetal heart in ultrasound video frames. Each frame is classified into three common standard views, e.g. four chamber view (4C), left ventricular outflow tract view (LVOT) and three vessel view (3V) captured in a typical ultrasound screening. Dong *et al.* [4] found the standard plane by fetal abdominal region localization in ultrasound using radial component model and selective search. Chen *et al.* [5] proposed an automatic framework based on deep learning to detect standard planes. The automatic framework achieved competitive performance and showed the potential and feasibility of deep learning for regions localization in ultrasound images. However, there are still lack of existing methods proposed under the clinical quality control criteria for quality assessment of fetal transthalamic plane in ultrasound images [6].

For quality control under the clinical criteria, the quality evaluation of the ultrasound images is scored via the number of the detected regions of important anatomical structures. The scores are given by comparing the detected region results with the bounding boxes annotated by doctors. Specifically, a standard transthalamic plane of fetal consists of 5 specific anatomical parts which can be clearly visualized, including lateral sulcus (LS), thalamus (T), choroid plexus (CP), cavum septi pellucidi (CSP) and third ventricle (TV). The ultrasound map and the specific pattern of the fetal head plane including transthalamic plane, transventricular plane, transcerebellar plane are shown in Fig. 1. However, the ultrasound images of these three planes are very similar and the doctors are confusing. In addition, there are remaining challenges for quality assessment of the ultrasound images due to the following limitations: (1) The quality of ultrasound images is often affected by noise; (2) The anatomical structure's area is scanned in different magnification levels; (3) The scanning angle and the fetal location are unstable due to the rotation of the anatomical structure; (4) There are high variations in shapes and sizes of the anatomical structures among the patients.

To solve the above-mentioned challenges, we propose a deep learning based method for quality assessment of the fetal transthalamic plane. Specifically, our proposed method is based on the popular faster region-based convolutional network (Faster R-CNN [7]) technique. The remarkable ability of Faster R-CNN has been demonstrated in effectively learning and extracting discriminative features from the training images. Faster R-CNN is able to simultaneously perform classification and detection tasks. First, the images and the annotated ground-truth boxes are fed into Faster R-CNN. Then, Faster R-CNN generates the bounding boxes and the scores to

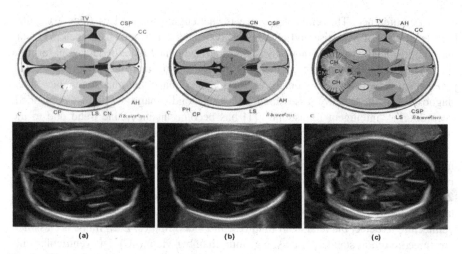

Fig. 1. The ultrasound map and the specific pattern of three fetal head plane. (a) transthalamic plane; (b) transventricular plane; (c) transcerebellar plane.

denote the detected regions and the quality of the detected regions, respectively. The output results are used to determine whether the ultrasound image is a standard plane. To the best of our knowledge, our proposed method is the first fully automatic deep learning based method for quality assessment of the fetal transthalamic plane in ultrasound images.

Overall, our contributions can be mainly highlighted as follows: (1) This is the first Faster R-CNN based method for the quality assessment of transthalamic plane of fetal; (2) The proposed framework could effectively assist doctors and reduce the workloads in the quality assessment of the transthalamic plane in ultrasound images; (3) Experimental results suggest that Fast R-CNN can be feasibly applied in many applications of ultrasound images. The proposed technique is generalized and can be easily extended to other medical image localization tasks.

2   Methodology

Figure 2 illustrates the framework of the proposed method for quality assessment of the fetal transthalamic plane. Faster R-CNN contains Fast R-CNN and RPN module. Images are cropped with a fixed-size of 224 × 224. The shared feature map, Fast R-CNN and RPN module of Faster R-CNN are explained in detail in this section.

2.1   Shared Feature Map

To achieve a fast detection while ensuring the accuracy of positioning results, the RPN module and Fast R-CNN [8] module share the first 5 convolutional layers of the convolutional neural network. However, the final effect and outputs of RPN and Fast R-CNN are different since the convolutional layers are modified in different ways.

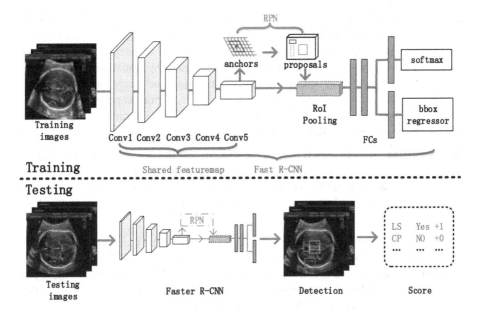

Fig. 2. The framework of our method based on Faster R-CNN.

At the same time, the feature map of the shared convolutional layer extraction must include the features required by both modules. This requirement cannot be easily obtained by just only using back propagation, which is in combination with the loss function optimization of the two modules. Fast R-CNN may not converge when the RPN could not provide fixed sizes of predicted bounding boxes.

To tackle the mentioned difficulties, Faster R-CNN learns the shared features through joint training and alternative optimization. Specifically, the pre-trained model of VGG16 is initialized and fine-tuned for training the RPN module. The generated bounding boxes are used as inputs to Fast R-CNN module. A separate detection network is then trained by Fast R-CNN. The pre-trained model of Fast R-CNN is the same as the pre-trained model of RPN module. However, these two networks are trained separately and do not share parameters. Next, the detection network is used to initialize the RPN training, but we fix the shared convolutional layer and only fine tune the RPN-specific layers. Then, we still keep the shared convolutional layer fixed and the RPN result is used to fine-tune the full connection layer of the Fast R-CNN module again. As a result, the two networks keep sharing the same convolutional layer until the end of the network training. Also, the detection and identification sets form a unified network.

2.2   Fast R-CNN Module

The structure of Fast R-CNN is designed based on R-CNN. In R-CNN, the processing steps (e.g., region proposal extraction, CNN features extraction, support vector machine (SVM) classification and box regression) are separated from each other that causes the training process hardly to optimize the network performance. By contrast, the training process of Fast R-CNN is executed in an end-to-end manner (except for the region proposal step). Fast R-CNN directly adds an region of interest (ROI) pooling layer, which is essentially equivalent to the simplification of spatial pyramid pooling (SPP). With ROI layer, Fast R-CNN convolutes an ultrasound image only once. Then, it extracts feature from the original image and locates its region proposal boxes, which greatly improves the speed of the network. Fast R-CNN eventually outputs the localization scores and the detected bounding-boxes simultaneously.

Base Network: Fast R-CNN is trained on VGG16 and the network is modified to be able to receive both input images and the annotated bounding boxes. Fast R-CNN preserves 13 convolutional layers and 4 max pooling layers of the VGG-16 architecture. In addition, the last fully connected layer and softmax of VGG16 are replaced by two sibling layers.

ROI Pooling Layer: The last max pooling layer of VGG16 is replaced by an ROI pooling layer to extract the fixed-length of feature vectors from the generated feature maps. Fast R-CNN is able to convolute an image only once. It extracts feature from the original image and locates its region proposal boxes, which boosts the speed of the network. Since the size of the ROI pooling input is varying, each pooling grid size needs to be designed, which ensures that the subsequent classification in each region can be normally preceded. For instance, the input size of a ROI is $h \times w$, the output size of the pooling is $H \times W$, and the size of each grid is designed as $h/H \times w/W$.

Loss Function: Two output layers of Fast R-CNN include the classification probability score prediction for each ROI region p, and the offset for each ROI region's coordinate $t^u = \left(t_x^u, t_y^u, t_w^u, t_h^u \right), 0 \le u \le U$, where U is the number of object classes. The loss function of Fast R-CNN is defined as follows:

$$L = \begin{cases} L_{cls}(p, u) + \lambda L_{loc}(t^u, v), & \text{if } u \text{ is a structure,} \\ L_{cls}(p, u), & \text{if } u \text{ is a background,} \end{cases} \tag{1}$$

where L_{cls} is the loss function of the classification, and L_{loc} is the loss function for the localization. It is worthy mentioned that we do not consider the loss function of the bounding boxes location if the classification result is misclassified as the background. The loss function of L_{cls} is defined as follows:

$$L_{cls}(p, u) = \log p_u, \tag{2}$$

where L_{loc} is also described as the difference between the predicted parameter t^u corresponding to the real classification and the true translation scaling parameter v. L_{loc} is defined as follows:

$$L_{loc}(t^u, v) = \sum_{i=1}^{4} g(t_i^u - v_i), \tag{3}$$

where g is the smooth deviation, which is more sensitive to the outlier. g is defined as

$$g(x) = \begin{cases} 0.5x^2, & |x| < 1, \\ |x| - 0.5, & otherwise. \end{cases} \tag{4}$$

2.3 RPN Module

The role of RPN module is to output the coordinates of a group of rectangular predicted bounding boxes. The implementation of RPN module did not slow down the training and detection process of the entire network because of the shared feature map. By taking the shared feature map as input of the RPN network, repetitive feature extraction is avoided and the calculation of regional attention is nearly cost-free. The RPN module performs convolution with a 3 × 3 sliding window on the incoming convolutional feature map and generate a 512-dimension feature matrix.

Then, RPN module also takes advantage of the principle of parallel output and accesses both branches after generating a 512-dimensional feature. The first branch is used to predict the upper left coordinates x, y, width w, and height h of the predicted bounding boxes corresponding to the central anchor points of the bounding boxes. For the diversity of predicted bounding boxes, the multi-scale method commonly is used in the RPN module. In order to obtain the more accurate predicted bounding boxes, the parameterizations of bounding box's coordinates are introduced. The second branch classifies the predicted bounding regions by the softmax classifier, which obtains a foreground bounding boxes and a background predicted bounding boxes (detection target is a foreground predicted bounding boxes). The last two branches converge at the FC layer, which is responsible for synthesizing the foreground predicted bounding box scores and the bounding box regression offsets, while removing the candidate boxes that are too small and out of bounds. In fact, the RPN module can get about 20,000 predicted bounding boxes, but there are many overlapping boxes. Here, a non-maximum suppression method is introduced to set the Intersection over Union (IOU) to a threshold of 0.7, i.e., preserving only predicted bounding boxes with local maximum score not exceeding 0.7. Finally, RPN module only passes 300 bounding boxes with higher score to the Fast R-CNN module. The RPN module not only simplifies the network input and improves the detection performance, but also enables the end-to-end training of the entire network, which is important for performance optimization.

3 Experiments

3.1 Dataset

The ultrasound images, which contain one single fetus, are collected from a local hospital. The gestation age of the fetus varies from 14 to 28 weeks. The most clearly visible images are selected in the second trimester. As a result, a total of 513 images which clearly visualize the 5 anatomical structures of LS, CP, T, CSP and TV are selected.

Due to the diversity of image sizes in the original dataset, the images are resized to 720 × 960 for further processing. Since the training for Faster R-CNN requires a large number of images, we increase the numbers and varieties of images by adopting a commonly used data augmentation method (e.g., random cropping, rotating and mirroring). As a result, a total of 4800 images are finally selected for training and the remaining 1153 images are used for testing. All the training and testing images are annotated and confirmed by an 8 years clinical experienced ultrasound doctor. All experiments are performed on a computer with CPU Inter Xeon E5-2680 @ 2.70 GHz, GPU NVIDIA Quadro K4000, and 128G of RAM.

3.2   Results

The setting of the training process is kept the same whenever possible for fair comparison. Recall (Rec), Precision (Prec) and Average Precision (AP) are used as performance evaluation metrics. We adopt 2 popular object detection methods including Fast R-CNN and Yolov2 [10] for performance comparisons. Table 1 summarizes the experimental results of each network. We observe that the detection results for single anatomical structure of the LS and CP are the best. This is because LS and CP have distinct contour, moderate size with high contrast and less surrounding interference. Another reason is that LS and CP classes contain more training samples than other classes, making the detection biased to detect these classes and misdetect other classes. The results of TV are quite low due to its blurry anatomical structure, small size, and structure similarity of other tissues.

Table 1. Comparison of the proposed method with other methods (%).

Method	Value	LS	CP	T	CSP	TV
Fast R-CNN	Rec	87.6	63.7	62.6	44.2	–
	Prec	84.7	57.0	60.8	29.3	–
	AP	70.6	36.3	39.5	19.8	–
YOLOv2	Rec	90.4	83.7	34.7	48.6	4.2
	Prec	99.6	97.2	79.9	94.1	85.2
	AP	90.3	82.9	30.3	46.9	3.6
Faster R-CNN (VGG16)	Rec	96.8	96.0	89.6	89.3	56.5
	Prec	96.6	96.7	77.1	94.6	72.8
	AP	**94.9**	**93.8**	**81.0**	**87.1**	**44.1**

Generally, the detection performance of Faster R-CNN is better than Fast R-CNN and Yolov2. In particular, Faster R-CNN has significantly improved the detection performance of TV. The running time per image from Fast R-CNN, YOLOv2, and Faster R-CNN is 2.7 s, 0.0006 s, and 0.27 s, respectively. Although the running time of Faster R-CNN is not the fastest, its speed still satisfies the clinical requirements.

Figure 3 shows the structure localization results using the proposed technique compared with other methods. The green, red, yellow, blue and green bounding boxes indicate the LS, CP, T, CSP and TV, respectively. As shown in Fig. 3, our method can simultaneously locate multiple anatomical structures in an ultrasound image and achieve the most superior localization results.

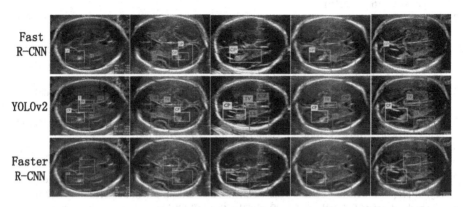

Fig. 3. The detection results of Fast R-CNN, YOLOv2, and Faster R-CNN (VGG16), respectively. The purple, yellow, cyan, red, and green boxes locate the lateral fissure, choroid plexus, thalamus, transparent compartment, and third ventricle, respectively. (Color figure online)

4 Conclusion

In this paper, we propose an automatic detection technique for quality assessment of fetal head in ultrasound images. We utilize Faster R-CNN to automatically locate five specific anatomical structures of the fetal transthalamic plane. Accordingly, the quality of the ultrasound image is scored and the standard plane is determined based on the number of detected regions. Experimental results demonstrate that it is feasible to employ deep learning for the quality assessment of fetal head ultrasound images. This technique can be also extended to many ultrasound images tasks. Our future work will tackle the existing problem of inhomogeneity of image contrast in ultrasound images, which will apply intensity enhancement method to enhance the contrast between the anatomical structures and the background. The clinical prior-knowledge will be utilized to achieve better detection and localization.

Acknowledgement. This work was supported partly by National Key Research and Develop Program (No. 2016YFC0104703).

References

1. Namburete, A., Xie, W., Yaqub, M., Zisserman, A., Noble, A.: Fully-automated alignment of 3D Fetal brain ultrasound to a canonical reference space using multi-task learning. Med. Image Anal. **46**, 1 (2018)
2. Li, J., et al.: Automatic fetal head circumference measurement in ultrasound using random forest and fast ellipse fitting. IEEE J. Biomed. Health Inf. **17**, 1–12 (2017)
3. Sundaresan, V., Bridge, C.P., Ioannou, C., Noble, J.A.: Automated characterization of the fetal heart in ultrasound images using fully convolutional neural networks. In: ISBI, pp. 671–674 (2017)
4. Ni, D., et al.: Standard plane localization in ultrasound by radial component model and selective search. Ultrasound Med. Biol. **40**, 2728–2742 (2014)
5. Chen, H., et al.: Standard plane localization in fetal ultrasound via domain transferred deep neural networks. IEEE J. Biomed. Health Inf. **19**, 1627–1636 (2015)
6. Li, S., et al.: Quality control of training prenatal ultrasound doctors in advanced training. Med. Ultrasound Chin. J. **6**, 14–17 (2009)
7. Ren, S., He, K., Girshick, R., Sun, J.: Faster R-CNN: towards real-time object detection with region proposal networks. IEEE Trans. Pattern Anal. Mach. Intell. **39**, 1137–1149 (2015)
8. Girshick, R.: Fast R-CNN. In: CVPR, pp. 1440–1448 (2015)

Recent Advances in Point-of-Care Ultrasound Using the *ImFusion Suite* for Real-Time Image Analysis

Oliver Zettinig[1(✉)], Mehrdad Salehi[1,2], Raphael Prevost[1], and Wolfgang Wein[1]

[1] ImFusion GmbH, Munich, Germany
zettinig@imfusion.de
[2] Computer Aided Medical Procedures, Technische Universität München, Munich, Germany

Abstract. Medical ultrasound is rapidly advancing both through more powerful hardware and software; in combination these allow the modality to become an ever more indispensable point-of-care tool. In this paper, we summarize some recent developments on the image analysis side that are enabled through the proprietary *ImFusion Suite* software and corresponding software development kit (SDK). These include 3D reconstruction of arbitrary untracked 2D US clips, image filtering and classification, speed-of-sound calibration and live acquisition parameter tuning in a visual servoing fashion.

1 Introduction

Today, a steadily increasing number of US device vendors dedicate their efforts on Point-of-Care Ultrasound (POCUS), including Philips[1], Butterfly[2], Clarius[3], UltraSee[4], and others. In general, these systems' development is hardware-driven and aims at introducing conventional scanning modes (B-mode, color Doppler) in previously inaccessible surroundings in the first place [1].

At the same time, significant work on improving non-point-of-care US has been presented in recent years [2]. Amongst them, three-dimensional (3D) US relying on external hardware tracking is already translating into clinical routine, enabling advanced live reconstruction of arbitrary anatomy [3]. Naturally,

---

O. Zettinig, M. Salehi and R. Prevost contributed equally to this paper.

[1] Philips Lumify®, Koninklijke Philips B.V., Netherlands, www.lumify.philips.com (accessed June 2018).

[2] Butterfly Network iQ®, Butterfly Network, Inc., NY, USA, www.butterflynetwork. com (accessed June 2018).

[3] Clarius®, Clarius Mobile Health, BC, Canada, www.clarius.me (accessed June 2018).

[4] Ultrasee Corp., CA, USA, ultraseecorp.com (accessed June 2018).

© Springer Nature Switzerland AG 2018
D. Stoyanov et al. (Eds.): POCUS 2018/BIVPCS 2018/CuRIOUS 2018/CPM 2018,
LNCS 11042, pp. 47–55, 2018.
https://doi.org/10.1007/978-3-030-01045-4_6

the trend to employ deep learning tools has not stopped short of US, exhibiting remarkable progress to segment challenging anatomies or classify suspicious lesions, as shown in the review by Litjens et al. [4] and references therein.

In liaison, these breakthroughs in terms of hardware and image processing allow us to look beyond conventional usage of US data. In this work, we summarize recent advances in POCUS and interventional US using innovative image analysis and machine learning technologies, which were implemented within our medical imaging framework *ImFusion Suite.*

For instance, very long 3D US scans facilitate automatic vessel mapping, cross-section and volume measurements as well as interventional treatment planning (available on an actual medical device now, see PIUR tUS[5]). Brain shift compensation based on multi-modal 3D US registration to pre-operative MR images enables accurate neuro-navigation, which has successfully been proven on real patients during surgery [5].

In the remainder of the paper, we start with a brief overview of the important features of our *ImFusion* software development kit (SDK) allowing for such developments and then highlight the following applications in greater detail: (i) Employing deep learning and optionally inertial measurement units (IMU), we have been able to show that 3D reconstruction is even possible without external tracking systems. (ii) For orthopedic surgery, precise bone surface segmentation facilitates intra-operative registration with sub-millimeter accuracy, in turn allowing for reliable surgical navigation. (iii) Last but not least, ultrasound uniquely allows to close the loop on the acquisition pipeline by actively influencing how the tissue is insonified and the image formed. We perform a tissue-specific speed-of-sound calibration, apply learning-based filtering to enhance image quality and optimally tune the acquisition parameters in real-time.

2   ImFusion SDK as Research Platform

A variety of open source C++ platforms and frameworks for medical imaging and navigation with US have evolved in the past, including 3D Slicer [6] with the SlicerIGT extension [7], the PLUS toolkit [8], CustusX [9], and more recently SUPRA [10]. All of these have a research focus, and have successfully helped to prototype novel algorithms and clinical workflows in the past, some with a very active development community striving for continuous improvement. Nevertheless, turning an algorithm from a research project into a user-friendly, certified medical product may be a long path.

Complementary to the above, we are presenting the *ImFusion Suite* & SDK, a platform for versatile medical image analysis research and product-grade software development. The platform is based on a set of proprietary core components, whereupon openly accessible plugins contributed by the research community can be developed. In this work, we emphasize the platform's capabilities to support academic researchers in rapid prototyping and translating scientific

---

[5] PIUR imaging GmbH, Vienna, Austria, www.piurimaging.com (accessed June 2018).

ideas to clinical studies and potential subsequent commercialization in the form of university spin-offs. The SDK has been employed by various groups around the world already [5,11–14].

It offers radiology workstation look and feel, ultra-fast DICOM loading, seamless CPU/OpenGL/OpenCL synchronization, advanced visualization, and various technology modules for specialized applications. In order to deal with real-time inputs such as ultrasound imaging or tracking sensors and other sensory information, the streaming sub-system is robust, thread-safe on both CPU and GPU, and easily extensible. Research users may script their algorithms using XML-based workspace configurations or a Python wrapper. Own plugins can be added using the C++ interface. In the context of dealing with 3D ultrasound, further key features that go beyond what is otherwise available include robust image-based calibration tools similar to [15], and various 3D compounding methods that allow for on-the-fly reconstruction of MPR cross-sections [16]. Last but not least, handling of tracking sensors include various synchronization, filtering and interpolation methods on the stream of homogeneous transformation matrices. Having all of the above readily available allows researchers to focus on advancing the state of the art with their key contribution, as demonstrated in the following examples.

3   3D POCUS Without External Tracking

Most POCUS systems are currently based on 2D ultrasound imaging, which greatly restricts the variety of clinical applications. While there exist systems enabling the acquisition of three-dimensional ultrasound data, they always come with drawbacks. 3D matrix-array ultrasound probes are very expensive and produce images with limited field-of-view and quality. On the other hand, optical or electro-magnetic tracking systems are expensive, not easily portable, or hinder usability by requiring a permanent line-of-sight. Finally, leveraging the inertial measurement units (IMU) that are embedded in most current US probes provides a good estimate of the probe orientation, but acceleration data is not accurate enough to compute its spatial position.

Therefore, in the past decades, there has been a significant effort in the research community to design a system that would not require additional and cumbersome hardware [18,19], yet allowing for 3D reconstruction with a freehand swept 2D probe. The standard approach for a purely image-based motion estimation was named *speckle decorrelation* since it exploits the frame-to-frame correlation of the speckle pattern present in US images. However, due to the challenging nature of the problem, even recent implementations of this approach have not reached an accuracy compatible with clinical requirements.

Once again, deep learning enabled a breakthrough by boosting the performance of image-based motion estimation. As we have shown in [17], it is possible to train a network to learn the 3D motion of the probe between two successive frames in an end-to-end fashion: the network takes the two frames as input and directly outputs the parameters of the translation and rotation of the probe

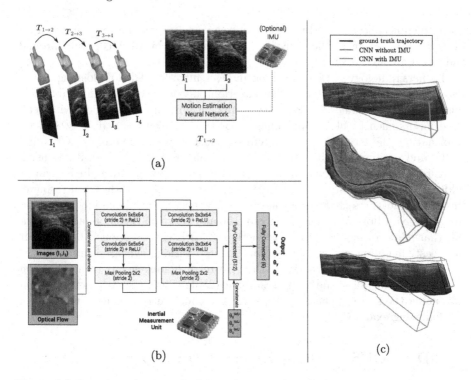

Fig. 1. (a) Overview of our method for a frame-to-frame trajectory estimation of the probe. (b) Architecture of the neural network at the core of the method. (c) Results of the reconstructed trajectories (without any external tracking) on several sweeps acquired with a complex motion. *From* [17], *modified.*

(see Fig. 1a and b). By applying such a network sequentially to a whole freehand sweep, we can reconstruct the complete trajectory of the probe and therefore compound the 2D frames into a high-resolution 3D volume. We also show that the IMU information can be embedded into the network to further improve the accuracy of the reconstruction. On a dataset of more than 700 sweeps, our approach yields trajectories with a median normalized drift of merely 5.2%, yielding unprecedentedly accurate length measurements with a median error of 3.4%. Example comparisons to ground truth trajectories are shown in Fig. 1c.

4   Ultrasound Image Analysis

A core feature of the *ImFusion* SDK consists of its capabilities for real-time image analysis. Provided that the employed US system allows for raw data access, the processing pipeline from live in-phase and quadrature (IQ) data regularly starts with demodulation, log-compression, scan-line conversion, and denoising.

Image Filtering. Instead of relying on conventional non-linear image filters, it is possible to use convolutional neural networks (CNNs) for denoising. Simple

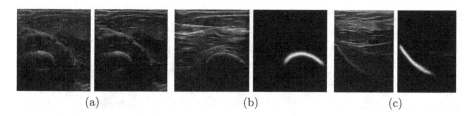

(a)   (b)   (c)

Fig. 2. (a) Raw B-mode image of volunteer forearm cross-section (*left*), and the result of the CNN-based denoising filter (*right*). **(b)(c)** Examples of automatic bone segmentations in various US images (different bones and acquisition settings), along with the neural network detection map. *From* [21], *modified*.

networks with U-net architecture [20] can be trained with l2-loss to perform a powerful, anatomy-independent noise reduction. Figure 2a depicts an exemplary B-mode image of a forearm in raw and filtered form. More complex, application-specific models could be used to emphasize a desired appearance, or to highlight suspicious lesions automatically.

Bone Surface Segmentation and Registration. As presented in [21], we have shown that the automatic segmentation of bone surfaces in US images is highly beneficial in Computer Assisted Orthopedic Surgeries (CAOS) and could replace X-ray fluoroscopy in various intra-operative scenarios. Specifically, a fully CNN was trained a set of labeled images, where the bone area has been roughly drawn by several users. Because the network turned out to be very reliable, simple thresholding and center pixel extraction between the maximum gradient and the maximum intensity proved sufficient to determine the bone surface line, see example results in Fig. 2b, c. Once a 3D point cloud of the bone surface was assembled using an external optical tracking system, pre-operative datasets such as CT or MRI can be registered by minimizing the point-to-surface error. An evaluation on 1382 US images from different volunteers, different bones (femur, tibia, patella, pelvis) and various acquisition settings yielded a median precision of 0.91 and recall of 0.94. On a human cadaver with fiducial markers for ground truth registration, the method achieved sub-millimetric surface registration errors and mean fiducial errors of 2.5 mm.

5   Speed-of-Sound Calibration

In conventional delay-sum US beamforming, speed-of-sound inconsistencies across tissues can distort the image along the scan-lines direction. The reason is that US machines assume a constant speed-of-sound for human tissue; however, the speed-of-sound varies in the human soft tissue with an approximate range of 150 m/s (Fig. 3a). To improve the spatial information quality, we have developed a fast speed-of-sound calibration method based on the bone surface detection algorithm outlined in the previous section.

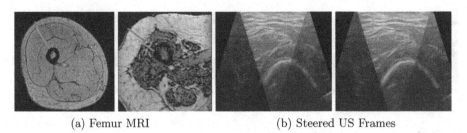

(a) Femur MRI   (b) Steered US Frames

Fig. 3. **(a)** The difference in fat-to-muscle ratio between two patients; red and green lines show the length of fat and muscle tissues. Considering the average speed-of-sound in human fat and muscle (1470 m/s and 1620 m/s), one can compute the average speed-of-sound for both images, resulting in 1590 m/s and 1530 m/s, respectively. At a depth of 6 cm, this difference can produce around 1 mm vertical shift in the structures. **(b)** Superimposed steered US images before (*left*) and after (*right*) the speed-of-sound calibration; red and green intensities are depicting the individual steered frames with angles of ±15°. Note the higher consistency of the bone in the right image. (Color figure online)

As presented in [21], two US steered frames with a positive and a negative angle are acquired in addition to the main image. Then, the bone surface is detected in the steered images and they are interpolated into one single frame. Wrong speed-of-sound causes both vertical and horizontal misplacements for the bone surface in the steered images. The correct speed-of-sound is estimated by maximizing the image similarity in the detected bone region captured from the different angles (Fig. 3b). This method is fast enough to facilitate real-time speed-of-sound compensation and hence to improve the spatial information extracted from US images during the POCUS procedures.

6   Acquisition Parameter Tuning

One last obstacle of a wider adoption of ultrasound is the inter-operator variability of the acquisition process itself. The appearance of the formed image indeed depends on a number of parameters (frequency, focus, dynamic range, brightness, etc.) whose tuning requires significant knowledge and experience. While we have already shown above that – thanks to deep learning – US image analysis algorithms can be made very robust to a sub-optimal tuning of such parameters, we can even go one step further and close the loop of the acquisition pipeline.

Just like standard cameras use face detection algorithm to adjust the focus plane and the exposure of a picture, we can leverage a real-time detection of the object of interest in the ultrasound frame to adjust the acquisition parameters automatically as shown in Fig. 4. Using machine learning to assess the image quality of an ultrasound image has already been proposed (e.g. [22]), but using a real-time detection allows to tailor our tuning of the parameters in an explicit and straightforward way.

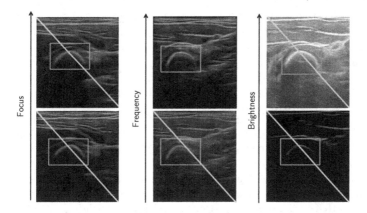

Fig. 4. Automatic tuning of the US acquisition parameters based on the real-time bone detection presented in Sect. 4, sub-optimal settings marked with red lines. (Color figure online)

More specifically, knowing the position of the object in the image allows us to directly set the focus plane of the ultrasound beams to the correct depth. It also enables us to adjust the frequency empirically: the shallower the object, the higher we can define the frequency (and vice versa). Finally, we can also choose an adequate brightness and dynamic range based on statistics within a region of interest that includes the target structure.

We believe such an algorithm could allow less experienced users to acquire ultrasound images with satisfactory quality, and therefore make the modality more popular for a larger number of clinical applications.

7   Conclusion

We have presented a number of advanced POCUS & interventional US applications through the *ImFusion Suite*. While many aspects of 3D ultrasound with and without external tracking have been thoroughly investigated by the community in the past, dealing with such data is by no means trivial, hence dedicated software was in our experience crucial to achieve such results.

Acknowledgments. This work was partially supported by H2020-FTI grant (number 760380) delivered by the European Union.

References

1. Campbell, S.J., Bechara, R., Islam, S.: Point-of-care ultrasound in the intensive care unit. Clin. Chest Med. **39**(1), 79–97 (2018)
2. Che, C., Mathai, T.S., Galeotti, J.: Ultrasound registration: a review. Methods **115**, 128–143 (2017)

3. Mozaffari, M.H., Lee, W.S.: Freehand 3-D ultrasound imaging: a systematic review. Ultrasound Med. Biol. **43**(10), 2099–2124 (2017)
4. Litjens, G., et al.: A survey on deep learning in medical image analysis. Med. Image Anal. **42**, 60–88 (2017)
5. Reinertsen, I., Iversen, D., Lindseth, F., Wein, W., Unsgård, G.: Intra-operative ultrasound based correction of brain-shift. In: Intraoperative Imaging Society Conference, Hanover, Germany (2017)
6. Kikinis, R., Pieper, S.D., Vosburgh, K.G.: 3D slicer: a platform for subject-specific image analysis, visualization, and clinical support. In: Jolesz, F. (ed.) Intraoperative Imaging and Image-Guided Therapy, pp. 277–289. Springer, New York (2014). https://doi.org/10.1007/978-1-4614-7657-3_19
7. Ungi, T., Lasso, A., Fichtinger, G.: Open-source platforms for navigated image-guided interventions. Med. Image Anal. **33**, 181–186 (2016)
8. Lasso, A., Heffter, T., Rankin, A., Pinter, C., Ungi, T., Fichtinger, G.: PLUS: open-source toolkit for ultrasound-guided intervention systems. IEEE Trans. Biomed. Eng. **61**(10), 2527–2537 (2014)
9. Askeland, C., et al.: CustusX: an open-source research platform for image-guided therapy. IJCARS **11**(4), 505–519 (2015)
10. Göbl, R., Navab, N., Hennersperger, C.: SUPRA: open source software defined ultrasound processing for real-time applications. Int. J. Comput. Assist. Radiol. Surg. **13**(6), 759–767 (2017)
11. Zettinig, O., et al.: 3D ultrasound registration-based visual servoing for neurosurgical navigation. IJCARS **12**(9), 1607–1619 (2017)
12. Riva, M., et al.: 3D intra-operative ultrasound and MR image guidance: pursuing an ultrasound-based management of brainshift to enhance neuronavigation. IJCARS **12**(10), 1711–1725 (2017)
13. Nagaraj, Y., Benedicks, C., Matthies, P., Friebe, M.: Advanced inside-out tracking approach for real-time combination of MRI and US images in the radio-frequency shielded room using combination markers. In: EMBC, pp. 2558–2561. IEEE (2016)
14. Şen, H.T., et al.: Cooperative control with ultrasound guidance for radiation therapy. Front. Robot. AI **3**, 49 (2016)
15. Wein, W., Khamene, A.: Image-based method for in-vivo freehand ultrasound calibration. In: SPIE Medical Imaging 2008, San Diego, February 2008
16. Karamalis, A., Wein, W., Kutter, O., Navab, N.: Fast hybrid freehand ultrasound volume reconstruction. In: Miga, M., Wong, I., Kenneth, H. (eds.) Proceedings of the SPIE, vol. 7261, pp. 726114–726118 (2009)
17. Prevost, R., et al.: 3D freehand ultrasound without external tracking using deep learning. Med. Image Anal. **48**, 187–202 (2018)
18. Prager, R.W., Gee, A.H., Treece, G.M., Cash, C.J., Berman, L.H.: Sensorless freehand 3-D ultrasound using regression of the echo intensity. Ultrasound Med. Biol. **29**(3), 437–446 (2003)
19. Gao, H., Huang, Q., Xu, X., Li, X.: Wireless and sensorless 3D ultrasound imaging. Neurocomputing **195**(C), 159–171 (2016)
20. Ronneberger, O., Fischer, P., Brox, T.: U-Net: convolutional networks for biomedical image segmentation. In: Navab, N., Hornegger, J., Wells, W.M., Frangi, A.F. (eds.) MICCAI 2015. LNCS, vol. 9351, pp. 234–241. Springer, Cham (2015). https://doi.org/10.1007/978-3-319-24574-4_28

21. Salehi, M., Prevost, R., Moctezuma, J.-L., Navab, N., Wein, W.: Precise ultrasound bone registration with learning-based segmentation and speed of sound calibration. In: Descoteaux, M., Maier-Hein, L., Franz, A., Jannin, P., Collins, D.L., Duchesne, S. (eds.) MICCAI 2017. LNCS, vol. 10434, pp. 682–690. Springer, Cham (2017). https://doi.org/10.1007/978-3-319-66185-8_77

22. El-Zehiry, N., Yan, M., Good, S., Fang, T., Zhou, S.K., Grady, L.: Learning the manifold of quality ultrasound acquisition. In: Mori, K., Sakuma, I., Sato, Y., Barillot, C., Navab, N. (eds.) MICCAI 2013. LNCS, vol. 8149, pp. 122–130. Springer, Heidelberg (2013). https://doi.org/10.1007/978-3-642-40811-3_16

Markerless Inside-Out Tracking for 3D Ultrasound Compounding

Benjamin Busam[1,2(✉)], Patrick Ruhkamp[1,2], Salvatore Virga[1],
Beatrice Lentes[1], Julia Rackerseder[1], Nassir Navab[1,3],
and Christoph Hennersperger[1]

[1] Computer Aided Medical Procedures, Technische Universität München,
Munich, Germany
salvo.virga@tum.de
[2] FRAMOS GmbH, Taufkirchen, Germany
{b.busam,p.ruhkamp}@framos.com
[3] Computer Aided Medical Procedures, Johns Hopkins University,
Baltimore, USA

Abstract. Tracking of rotation and translation of medical instruments plays a substantial role in many modern interventions and is essential for 3D ultrasound compounding. Traditional external optical tracking systems are often subject to line-of-sight issues, in particular when the region of interest is difficult to access. The introduction of inside-out tracking systems aims to overcome these issues. We propose a marker-less tracking system based on visual SLAM to enable tracking of ultrasound probes in an interventional scenario. To achieve this goal, we mount a miniature multi-modal (mono, stereo, active depth) vision system on the object of interest and relocalize its pose within an adaptive map of the operating room. We compare state-of-the-art algorithmic pipelines and apply the idea to transrectal 3D ultrasound (TRUS). Obtained volumes are compared to reconstruction using a commercial optical tracking system as well as a robotic manipulator. Feature-based binocular SLAM is identified as the most promising method and is tested extensively in challenging clinical environments and for the use case of prostate US biopsies.

Keywords: 3D ultrasound imaging · Line-of-sight avoidance
Visual inside-out tracking · SLAM · Computer assisted interventions

1 Introduction

Tracking of medical instruments and tools is required for various systems in medical imaging, as well as computer aided interventions. Especially for medical applications such as 3D ultrasound compounding, accurate tracking is an important requirement, however often comes with severe drawbacks impacting the medical workflow. Mechanical tracking systems can provide highly precise

© Springer Nature Switzerland AG 2018
D. Stoyanov et al. (Eds.): POCUS 2018/BIVPCS 2018/CuRIOUS 2018/CPM 2018,
LNCS 11042, pp. 56–64, 2018.
https://doi.org/10.1007/978-3-030-01045-4_7

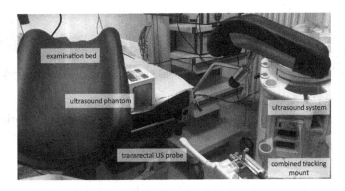

Fig. 1. Interventional setup for fusion biopsy. Clinical settings are often characterized by cluttered setups with tools and equipment around the examination bed. While such environments are challenging for outside-in tracking, they can provide a rich set of features for SLAM-based inside-out tracking.

tracking through a kinematic chain [1]. These systems often require bulky and expensive equipment, which cannot be adapted to a clinical environment where high flexibility needs to be ensured. In contrast to that, electromagnetic tracking is flexible in its use, but limited to comparably small work spaces and can interfere with metallic objects in proximity to the target, reducing the accuracy [2].

Optical tracking systems (OTS) enjoy widespread use as they do not have these disadvantages. Despite favourable spatial accuracy under optimal conditions, respective systems suffer from constraints by the required line-of-sight. Robust marker based methods such as [3] address this problem and work even if the target is only partly visible. However, the marker-visibility issue is further complicated for imaging solutions relying on tracking systems, with prominent examples being freehand SPECT [4] as well as freehand 3D ultrasound [5].

Aiming at both accurate and flexible systems for 3D imaging, a series of developments have been proposed recently. Inside-out tracking for collaborative robotic imaging [6] proposes a marker-based approach using infrared cameras, however, not resolving line-of-sight issues. A first attempt at making use of localized features employs tracking of specific skin features for estimation of 3D poses [7] in 3D US imaging. While this work shows promising results, it is constrained to the specific anatomy at hand.

In contrast to previous works, our aim is to provide a generalizable tracking approach without requiring a predefined or application-specific set of features while being easy to setup even for novice users. With the recent advent of advanced miniaturized camera systems, we evaluate an inside-out tracking approach solely relying on features extracted from image data for pose tracking (Fig. 1).

For this purpose, we propose the use of visual methods for simultaneously mapping the scenery and localizing the system within it. This is enabled by building up a map from characteristic structures within the previously unknown scene observed by a camera, which is known as SLAM [8]. Different image

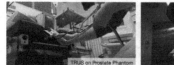

Fig. 2. 3D TRUS volume acquisition of prostate phantom. An inside-out camera is mounted on a transrectal US transducer together with a rigid marker for an outside-in system in the prostate biopsy OR. The consecutive images show the relevant extracted data for the considered SLAM methods.

modalities can be used for visual SLAM and binocular stereo possesses many benefits compared to monocular vision or active depth sensors.

On this foundation, we propose a flexible inside-out tracking approach relying on image features and poses retrieved from SLAM. We evaluate different methods in direct comparison to a commercial tracking solution and ground truth, and show an integration for freehand 3D US imaging as one potential use-case. The proposed prototype is the first proof of concept for SLAM-based inside-out tracking for interventional applications, applied here to 3D TRUS as shown in Fig. 2. The novelty of pointing the camera away from the patient into the quasi-static room while constantly updating the OR map enables advantages in terms of robustness, rotational accuracy and line-of-sight problem avoidance. Thus, no hardware relocalization of external outside-in systems is needed, partial occlusion is handled with wide-angle lenses and the method copes with dynamic environmental changes. Moreover, it paves the path for automatic multi-sensor alignment through a shared common map while maintaining an easy installation by clipping the sensor to tools.

2   Methods

For interventional imaging and specifically for the case of 3D ultrasound, the goal is to provide rigid body transformations of a desired target with respect to a common reference frame. This way, we denote $^{B}\mathbf{T}_A$ as transformation A to B. On this foundation, the transformation $^{W}\mathbf{T}_{US}$ from the ultrasound image (US) should be indicated in a desired world coordinate frame (W). For the case of inside-out based tracking - and in contrast to outside-in approaches - the ultrasound probe is rigidly attached to the camera system, providing the desired relation to the world reference frame

$$^{W}\mathbf{T}_{US} = {}^{W}\mathbf{T}_{RGB} \cdot {}^{RGB}\mathbf{T}_{US}, \tag{1}$$

where $^{W}\mathbf{T}_{RGB}$ is retrieved from tracking. The static transformation $^{RGB}\mathbf{T}_{US}$ can be obtained with a conventional 3D US calibration method [9].

Inside-out tracking is proposed on the foundation of a miniature camera setup as described in Sect. 3. The setup provides different image modalities for the visual SLAM. Monocular SLAM is not suitable for our needs, since it needs an appropriate translation without rotation within the first frames for proper initialization and suffers from drift due to accumulating errors over time. Furthermore, the absolute scale of the reconstructed map and the trajectory is unknown due to the arbitrary baseline induced by the non-deterministic initialization for finding a suitable translation. Relying on the depth data from the sensor would not be sufficient for the desired tracking accuracy, due to noisy depth information. A stereo setup can account for absolute scale by a known fixed baseline and movements with rotations only can be accounted for since matched feature points can be triangulated for each frame.

For the evaluations we run experiments with publicly available SLAM methods for better reproducibility and comparability. ORB-SLAM2 [8] is used as state-of-the-art feature based method. The well-known direct methods [10,11] are not eligible due to the restriction to monocular cameras. We rely on the recent publicly available[1] stereo implementation of Direct Sparse Odometry (DSO) [12].

The evaluation is performed with the coordinate frames depicted in Fig. 3. The intrinsic camera parameters of the involved monocular and stereo cameras (RGB, IR1, IR2) are estimated as proposed by [13]. For the rigid transformation from the robotic end effector to the inside-out camera, we use the hand-eye calibration algorithm of Tsai-Lenz [14] in eye-on-hand variant implemented in ViSP [15] and the eye-on-base version to obtain the rigid transformation from the optical tracking system to the robot base. To calibrate the ultrasound image plane with respect to the different tracking systems, we use the open source PLUS ultrasound toolkit [16] and provide a series of correspondence pairs using a tracked stylus pointer.

3   Experiments and Validation

To validate the proposed tracking approach, we first evaluate the tracking accuracy, followed by a specific analysis for the suitability to 3D ultrasound imaging. We use a KUKA iiwa (KUKA Roboter GmbH, Augsburg, Germany) 7 DoF robotic arm to gather ground truth tracking data which guarantees a positional reproducibility of ± 0.1 mm. To provide a realistic evaluation, we also utilize an optical infrared-based outside-in tracking system (Polaris Vicra, Northern Digital Inc., Waterloo, Canada). Inside-out tracking is performed with the Intel RealSense Depth Camera D435 (Mountain View, US), providing RGB and infrared stereo data in a portable system (see Fig. 3). Direct and feature based SLAM methods for markerless inside-out tracking are compared and evaluated against marker based optical inside-out tracking with ArUco [17] markers (16×16 cm) and classical optical outside-in tracking. For a quantitative analysis, a combined marker with an optical target and a miniature vision sensor is attached to the robot end effector. The robot is controlled using the Robot Operating System (ROS) while the camera acquisition is done on a separate machine

---

[1] https://github.com/JiatianWu/stereo-dso, Horizon Robotics, Inc. Beijing, China, Authors: Wu, Jiatian; Yang, Degang; Yan, Qinrui; Li, Shixin.

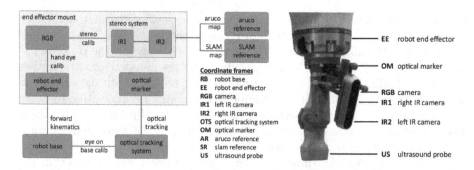

Fig. 3. System architecture and coordinate frames. Shown are all involved coordinate reference frames to evaluate the system performance (**left**) as well as the specific ultrasound mount used for validation, integrating optical and camera-based tracking with one attachable target (**right**).

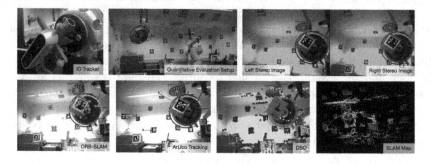

Fig. 4. Quantitative evaluation setup. The first row illustrates the operating room where the quantitative analysis is performed together with the inside-out stereo view. The second row depicts various calculated SLAM information necessary to create the map.

using the intel RealSense SDK[2]. The pose of the RGB camera and the tracking target are communicated via TCP/IP with a publicly available library[3]. The images are processed on an intel Core i7-6700 CPU, 64bit, 8 GB RAM running Ubuntu 14.04. We use the same constraints as in a conventional TRUS. Thus, the scanning time, covered volume and distance of the tracker is directly comparable and the error analysis reflects this specific procedure with all involved components. Figure 4 shows the clinical environment for the quantitative evaluation together with the inside-out view and the extracted image information for the different SLAM methods.

---

[2] https://github.com/IntelRealSense/librealsense.
[3] https://github.com/IFL-CAMP/simple.

3.1 Tracking Accuracy

To evaluate the tracking accuracy, we use the setup described above and acquire a series of pose sequences. The robot is programmed to run in gravity compensation mode such that it can be directly manipulated by a human operator. The forward kinematics of a robotic manipulator are used as ground truth (GT) for the actual movement.

To allow for error evaluation, we transform all poses of the different tracking systems in the joint coordinate frame coinciding at the RGB-camera of the end effector mount (see Fig. 3 for an overview of all reference frames)

$$^{RGB}\mathbf{T}_{RB} = {}^{RGB}\mathbf{T}_{EE} \cdot {}^{EE}\mathbf{T}_{RB} \tag{2}$$

$$^{RGB}\mathbf{T}_{SR} = {}^{RGB}\mathbf{T}_{EE} \cdot {}^{EE}\mathbf{T}_{RB} \cdot {}^{RB}\mathbf{T}_{IR1,0} \cdot {}^{IR1,0}\mathbf{T}_{SR} \tag{3}$$

$$^{RGB}\mathbf{T}_{AR} = {}^{RGB}\mathbf{T}_{EE} \cdot {}^{EE}\mathbf{T}_{RB} \cdot {}^{RB}\mathbf{T}_{IR1,0} \cdot {}^{IR1,0}\mathbf{T}_{AR} \tag{4}$$

$$^{RGB}\mathbf{T}_{OTS} = {}^{RGB}\mathbf{T}_{EE} \cdot {}^{EE}\mathbf{T}_{RB} \cdot {}^{RB}\mathbf{T}_{OTS} \cdot {}^{OTS}\mathbf{T}_{OM}, \tag{5}$$

providing a direct way to compare the optical tracking system (OTS), to SLAM-based methods (SR), and the ArUco-based tracking (AR).

In overall, 5 sequences were acquired with a total of 8698 poses. The pose error for all compared system is indicated in Fig. 5, where the translation error is given by the RMS of the residuals compared with the robotic ground truth while the illustrated angle error gives angular deviation of the rotation axis. From the results it can be observed that optical tracking provides the best results, with translation errors of 1.90 ± 0.53 mm, followed by 2.65 ± 0.74 mm for ORB-SLAM and 3.20 ± 0.96 for DSO, ArUco with 5.73 ± 1.44 mm. Interestingly, the SLAM-based methods provide better results compared to OTS, with errors of $1.99 \pm 1.99°$ for ORB-SLAM, followed by $3.99 \pm 3.99°$ for DSO, respectively. OTS estimates result in errors of $8.43 \pm 6.35°$, and ArUco orientations are rather noisy with $29.75 \pm 48.92°$.

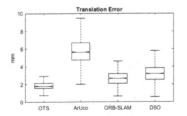 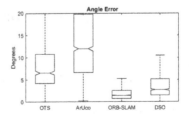

Fig. 5. Comparison of tracking error. Shown are translational and rotational errors compared to ground truth for all evaluated systems.

3.2 Markerless Inside-Out 3D Ultrasound

On the foundation of favourable tracking characteristics, we evaluate the performance of a markerless inside-out 3D ultrasound system by means of image quality and reconstruction accuracy for a 3D US compounding. For imaging, the tracking mount shown in Fig. 3 is integrated with a 128 elements linear transducer (CPLA12875, 7 MHz) connected to a cQuest Cicada scanner (Cephasonics, CA, USA). For data acquisition, a publicly available real-time framework is employed.[4] We perform a sweep acquisition, comparing OTS outside-in tracking with the proposed inside-out method and evaluate the quality of the reconstructed data while we deploy [18] for temporal pose synchronization. Figure 6 shows a qualitative comparison of the 3D US compoundings for the same sweep with the different tracking methods.[5]

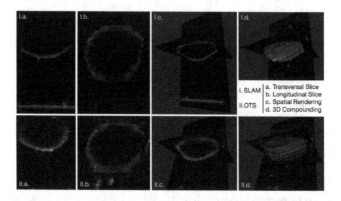

Fig. 6. Visualization of 3D US compounding quality. Shown are longitudinal and transversal slices as well as a 3D rendering of the resulting reconstructed 3D data from a tracked ultrasound acquisition of a ball phantom for the proposed tracking using ORB-SLAM in comparison with a commercial outside-in OTS. The structure appears spherically while the rotational accuracy advantage of ORB-SLAM causes a smoother rendering surface and a more clearly defined phantom boundary in the computed slices.

4   Discussion and Conclusion

From our evaluation, it appears that ArUco markers are viable only for approximate positioning within a room rather than accurate tracking. Our proposed inside-out approach shows valuable results compared to standard OTS and even outperforms the outside-in system in terms of rotational accuracy. These findings concur with assumptions based on the camera system design, as small rotations close to the optical principal point of the camera around any axis will lead to

---

[4] https://github.com/IFL-CAMP/supra.
[5] A video analysis of the method can be found here: https://youtu.be/SPy5860K49Q.

severe changes in the viewing angle, which can visually be described as inside-out rotation leverage effect.

One main advantage of the proposed methods is with respect to usability in practice. By not relying on specific markers, there is no need for setting up an external system or a change in setup during procedures. Additionally, we can avoid line-of-sight problems, and potentially allow for highly accurate tracking even for complete rotations around the camera axis without loosing tracking. This is in particular interesting for applications that include primarily rotation such as transrectal prostate fusion biopsy. Besides the results above, our proposed method is capable of orientating itself within an unknown environment by mapping its surrounding from the beginning of the procedure. This mapping is build up from scratch without the necessity of any additional calibration. Our tracking results for a single sensor also suggest further investigation towards collaborative inside-out tracking with multiple systems at the same time, orientating themselves within a global map as common reference frame.

References

1. Hennersperger, C., et al.: Towards MRIs-based autonomous robotic US acquisitions: a first feasibility study. MI **36**(2), 538–548 (2017)
2. Kral, F., Puschban, E.J., Riechelmann, H., Freysinger, W.: Comparison of optical and electromagnetic tracking for navigated lateral skull base surgery. IJMRCAS **9**(2), 247–252 (2013)
3. Busam, B., Esposito, M., Che'Rose, S., Navab, N., Frisch, B.: A stereo vision approach for cooperative robotic movement therapy. In: ICCVW, pp. 127–135 (2015)
4. Heuveling, D., Karagozoglu, K., Van Schie, A., Van Weert, S., Van Lingen, A., De Bree, R.: Sentinel node biopsy using 3D lymphatic mapping by freehand spect in early stage oral cancer: a new technique. CO **37**(1), 89–90 (2012)
5. Fenster, A., Downey, D.B., Cardinal, H.N.: Three-dimensional ultrasound imaging. Phys. Med. Biol. **46**(5), R67 (2001)
6. Esposito, M., et al.: Cooperative robotic gamma imaging: enhancing US-guided needle biopsy. In: Navab, N., Hornegger, J., Wells, W.M., Frangi, A.F. (eds.) MICCAI 2015. LNCS, vol. 9350, pp. 611–618. Springer, Cham (2015). https://doi.org/10.1007/978-3-319-24571-3_73
7. Sun, S.-Y., Gilbertson, M., Anthony, B.W.: Probe localization for freehand 3D ultrasound by tracking skin features. In: Golland, P., Hata, N., Barillot, C., Hornegger, J., Howe, R. (eds.) MICCAI 2014. LNCS, vol. 8674, pp. 365–372. Springer, Cham (2014). https://doi.org/10.1007/978-3-319-10470-6_46
8. Mur-Artal, R., Tardós, J.D.: ORB-SLAM2: an open-source slam system for monocular, stereo, and RGB-D cameras. TR **33**(5), 1255–1262 (2017)
9. Hsu, P.W., Prager, R.W., Gee, A.H., Treece, G.M.: Freehand 3D ultrasound calibration: a review. In: Sensen, C.W., Hallgrímsson, B. (eds.) Advanced Imaging in Biology and Medicine, pp. 47–84. Springer, Heidelberg (2009). https://doi.org/10.1007/978-3-540-68993-5_3
10. Engel, J., Schöps, T., Cremers, D.: LSD-SLAM: large-scale direct monocular SLAM. In: Fleet, D., Pajdla, T., Schiele, B., Tuytelaars, T. (eds.) ECCV 2014. LNCS, vol. 8690, pp. 834–849. Springer, Cham (2014). https://doi.org/10.1007/978-3-319-10605-2_54

11. Engel, J., Koltun, V., Cremers, D.: Direct sparse odometry. PAMI (2018)
12. Wang, R., Schwörer, M., Cremers, D.: Stereo DSO: large-scale direct sparse visual odometry with stereo cameras. In: ICCV (2017)
13. Zhang, Z.: A flexible new technique for camera calibration. PAMI **22**(11), 1330–1334 (2000)
14. Tsai, R.Y., Lenz, R.K.: A new technique for fully autonomous and efficient 3D robotics hand/eye calibration. TRA **5**(3), 345–358 (1989)
15. Marchand, É., Spindler, F., Chaumette, F.: Visp for visual servoing: a generic software platform with a wide class of robot control skills. RAM **12**(4), 40–52 (2005)
16. Lasso, A., Heffter, T., Rankin, A., Pinter, C., Ungi, T., Fichtinger, G.: Plus: open-source toolkit for ultrasound-guided intervention systems. BE **61**(10), 2527–2537 (2014)
17. Garrido-Jurado, S., noz Salinas, R.M., Madrid-Cuevas, F., Marín-Jiménez, M.: Automatic generation and detection of highly reliable fiducial markers under occlusion. PR **47**(6), 2280–2292 (2014)
18. Busam, B., Esposito, M., Frisch, B., Navab, N.: Quaternionic upsampling: Hyperspherical techniques for 6 DoF pose tracking. In: 3DV, IEEE (2016) 629–638

Ultrasound-Based Detection of Lung Abnormalities Using Single Shot Detection Convolutional Neural Networks

Sourabh Kulhare[1]([✉]), Xinliang Zheng[1], Courosh Mehanian[1],
Cynthia Gregory[2], Meihua Zhu[2], Kenton Gregory[1,2], Hua Xie[2],
James McAndrew Jones[2], and Benjamin Wilson[1]

[1] Intellectual Ventures Laboratory, Bellevue, WA 98007, USA
skulhare@intven.com
[2] Oregon Health Sciences University, Portland, OR 97239, USA

Abstract. Ultrasound imaging can be used to identify a variety of lung pathologies, including pneumonia, pneumothorax, pleural effusion, and acute respiratory distress syndrome (ARDS). Ultrasound lung images of sufficient quality are relatively easy to acquire, but can be difficult to interpret as the relevant features are mostly non-structural and require expert interpretation. In this work, we developed a convolutional neural network (CNN) algorithm to identify five key lung features linked to pathological lung conditions: B-lines, merged B-lines, lack of lung sliding, consolidation and pleural effusion. The algorithm was trained using short ultrasound videos of *in vivo* swine models with carefully controlled lung conditions. Key lung features were annotated by expert radiologists and snonographers. Pneumothorax (absence of lung sliding) was detected with an Inception V3 CNN using simulated M-mode images. A single shot detection (SSD) framework was used to detect the remaining features. Our results indicate that deep learning algorithms can successfully detect lung abnormalities in ultrasound imagery. Computer-assisted ultrasound interpretation can place expert-level diagnostic accuracy in the hands of low-resource health care providers.

Keywords: Lung ultrasound · Deep learning · Convolutional neural networks

1 Introduction

Ultrasound imaging is a versatile and ubiquitous imaging technology in modern healthcare systems. Ultrasound enables skilled sonographers to diagnose a diverse set of conditions and can guide a variety of interventions. Low cost ultrasound systems are becoming widely available, many of which are portable and have user-friendly touch displays. As ultrasound becomes more available and easier to operate, the limiting factor for adoption of diagnostic ultrasound will become the lack of training in interpreting images rather than the cost and complexity of ultrasound hardware. In remote settings like small health centers, combat medicine, and developing-world health care systems, the lack of experienced radiologists and skilled sonographers is already a key limiting factor for the effectiveness of ultrasound imaging. Recent advances in artificial

© Springer Nature Switzerland AG 2018
D. Stoyanov et al. (Eds.): POCUS 2018/BIVPCS 2018/CuRIOUS 2018/CPM 2018,
LNCS 11042, pp. 65–73, 2018.
https://doi.org/10.1007/978-3-030-01045-4_8

intelligence provide a potential route to improve access to ultrasound diagnostics in remote settings. State of the art computer vision algorithms such as convolutional neural networks have demonstrated performance matching that of humans on a variety of image interpretation tasks [1].

In this work, we demonstrate the feasibility of computer-assisted ultrasound diagnosis by using a CNN-based algorithm to identify abnormal pulmonary conditions. Ultrasound in most cases does not show any structural information from within the lung due to the high impedance contrast between the lung, which is mostly air, and the surrounding soft tissue. Despite this, lung ultrasound has gained popularity in recent years as a technique to detect pulmonary conditions such as pneumothorax, pneumonia, pleural effusion, pulmonary edema, and ARDS [2, 3]. Skilled sonographers can perform these tasks if they have been trained to find the structural features and non-structural artifacts correlated with disease. These include abstract features such as A-lines, B-lines, air bronchograms, and lung sliding. Pleural line is defined in ultrasound as a thin echogenic line at the interface between the superficial soft tissues and the air in the lung. A-line is a horizontal artifact indicating a normal lung surface. The B-line is an echogenic, coherent, wedge-shaped signal with a narrow origin in the near field of the image. Figure 1 shows examples of ultrasound lung images.

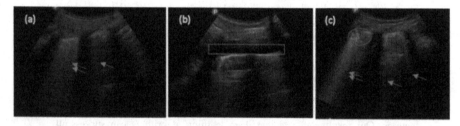

Fig. 1. Ultrasound images from swine modeling lung pathologies that demonstrate (a) single (single arrow) and merged B-lines (double arrow), (b) pleural effusion (box), and (c) single and merged B-lines along with consolidation (circle).

Lung ultrasound is an ideal target for computer-assisted diagnosis because imaging the lung is relatively straightforward. The lungs are easy to locate in the thorax and precise probe placement and orientation is not necessary to visualize key features. By selecting a target that is relatively easy to image but complicated to interpret, we maximize the potential benefit of the algorithm to an unskilled user.

Computer processing of ultrasound images is a well-established field. Most methods focus on tools that assist skilled users with metrology, segmentation, or tasks that expert operators perform inconsistently, unaided [4]. Methods for detecting B-lines have previously been reported [5–7]. A recent survey [8] outlines deep learning work on ultrasound lesion detection but there has been less work on consolidation and effusion. Other examples include segmentation and measurement of muscle and bones [9], carotid artery [10], and fetus orientation [11]. Note that while these efforts utilize CNNs, their goal is segmentation and metrology, as opposed to computer–assisted diagnosis.

To show the effectiveness of CNN-based computer vision algorithms for interpreting lung ultrasound images, this work leverages swine models with various lung pathologies, imaged with a handheld ultrasound system. We include an overview of the swine models and image acquisition and annotation procedures. We provide a description of our algorithm and its performance on swine lung ultrasound images. Our detection framework is based on single shot detection (SSD) [12], an efficient, state-of-the-art deep learning system suitable for embedded devices such as smart phones and tablets.

2 Approach

2.1 Animal Model, Data Collection and Annotation

All animal studies and ultrasound imaging were performed at Oregon Health & Science University (OHSU), following Institutional Animal Care and Use Committee (IACUC) and Animal Care and Use Review Office (ACURO) approval. Ultrasound data from swine lung pathology models were captured for both normal and abnormal lungs. Normal lung features included pleural lines and A-lines. Abnormal lung features included B-lines (single and merged), pleural effusion, pneumothorax, and consolidation. Models of 3 different lung pathologies were used to generate ultrasound data with one or more target features. For normal lung data collection (i.e. pleural line and A-line data collection), all animals were scanned prior to induction of lung pathology. For pneumothorax and pleural effusion ultrasound features, swine underwent percutaneous thoracic puncture of one hemithorax followed by injection of air and infusion with saline into the pleural space of the other hemithorax, respectively. For consolidation, single and merged B-line ultrasound features, in separate swine, acute respiratory distress syndrome (ARDS) was induced by inhalation of nebulized lipopolysaccharide. Examples of ultrasound images acquired from the animal studies are shown in Figs. 1 and 2.

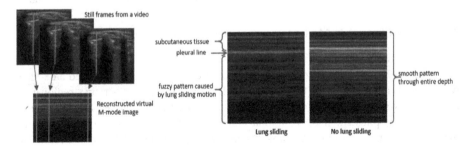

Fig. 2. Reconstruction of simulated M-mode images (left) and examples images (right).

Ultrasound data were acquired using a Lumify handheld system with a C5-2 broadband curved array transducer (Philips, Bothell, WA, USA). All images were acquired after selecting the Lumify app's lung preset. Per the guidelines for point-of-care lung ultrasound [13], the swine chest area was divided into eight zones. For each zone, at least two 3-s videos were collected at a frame rate of approximately 20 per second. One exam was defined as the collection of videos from all eight zones at each time point. Therefore, at least 16 videos were collected in each exam. For each swine, the lung pathology was induced incrementally and therefore, multiple exams were performed on each swine. Approximately 100 exams were performed with 2,200 videos collected in total. Lung ultrasound experts annotated target features frame-by-frame using a custom Matlab-based annotation tool.

2.2   Data Pre-processing

Input data for pre-processing consisted of either whole videos or video frames (images). Frame-level data was used to locate A-lines, single B-lines, merged B-lines, pleural line, pleural effusion, and consolidation. Video-level data was used for representation of pneumothorax. Raw ultrasound data collected from a curvilinear probe take the form of a polar coordinate image. These raw data were transformed from polar coordinates to Cartesian, which served to eliminate angular variation among B-lines and accelerate learning. The transformed images were cropped to remove uninformative data, such as dark borders and text, resulting in images with a resolution of 801×555 pixels.

Video data were similarly transformed to Cartesian coordinates. Each transformed video was used to generate simulated M-mode images. An M-mode image is a trace of a vertical line (azimuthal, in the original polar image) over time. The vertical sum threshold-based method [7] was used to detect intercostal spaces. Each intercostal space was sampled to generate ten M-mode images at equally spaced horizontal locations.

Ultrasound video of a healthy lung displays lung sliding, caused by the relative movement of parietal and visceral pleura during respiration. This can readily be observed in M-mode images, where there is a transition to a "seashore" pattern below the pleural line. Pneumothorax prevents observation of the relative pleural motion and causes the M-mode image to appear with uniform horizontal lines as shown in Fig. 2.

2.3   Single Shot CNN Model for Image-Based Lung Feature Detection

Single Shot Detector (SSD) is an extension of the family of regional convolutional neural networks (R-CNNs) [14–16]. Previous object detection methods used a de-facto two network approach, with the first network responsible for generating region proposals followed by a CNN to classify each proposal into target classes. SSD is a single network that applies small convolutional filters (detection filters) to the output feature maps of a base network to predict object category scores and bounding box offsets. The convolutional filters are applied to feature maps at multiple spatial scales to enable detection of objects of various sizes. Furthermore, multiple filters representing default bounding boxes of various aspect ratios are applied at each spatial location to detect objects of varying shapes. This architecture renders SSD an efficient and accurate object detection framework [17], making it a suitable choice for on-device inference tasks. Figure 3 provides an overview of the SSD architecture. Details can be found in [12].

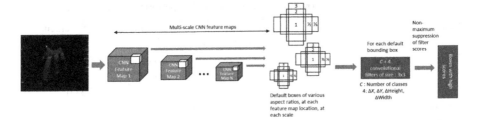

Fig. 3. SSD network schematic

Training. Each detection filter in SSD corresponds to a default bounding box at a particular location, at a particular scale, and aspect ratio. Prior to training, each ground truth bounding box is matched against the default bounding box with maximum Jaccard overlap. It is also matched against any default bounding box with Jaccard overlap greater than a threshold (usually 0.5). Thus, each ground truth box may be matched to more than one default box, which makes the learning problem smoother. The training objective of SSD is to minimize an overall loss that is a weighted sum of localization loss and confidence loss. Localization loss is Smooth L1 loss between location parameters of the predicted box and the ground truth box. Confidence loss is the softmax over multiple class confidences for each predicted box. We used horizontal flip, random crop, scale, and object box displacement as augmentations for training the lung features CNN models. For training the lung sliding model, we used Gaussian blur, random pixel intensity and contrast enhancement augmentations.

Hyperparameters. We use six single-class SSD networks as opposed to a multi-class network because the training data is small and unbalanced. Pleural lines and A-lines are abundant as they are normal lung features, whereas pathological lung features are rare. Furthermore, pleural line and pleural effusion features are in close proximity, thus there is significant overlap between their bounding boxes. Closely located features, combined with an unbalanced, small training set compromises performance when trained on multi-class SSD. We plan to address these issues in future work.

The train and test set sizes for each detection model are shown in Table 1. Feature models were trained for 300k iterations with batch size of 24, momentum 0.9, and initial learning rate of 0.004 (piece-wise constant learning rate that is reduced by 0.95 after every 80k iterations). We used the following aspect ratios for default boxes: 1, 2, 3, 1/2, 1/3, and 1/4. The base SSD network, Inception V2 [18], started with pre-trained ImageNet [19] weights and was fine-tuned for lung feature detection. The training process required 2–3 days per feature with the use of one GeForce GTX 1080Ti graphics card.

2.4 Inception V3 Architecture for Video-Based Lung Sliding Detection

Lung sliding was detected using virtual M-mode images that were generated by the process described in Sect. 2.2. We trained a binary classifier based on the Inception V3 CNN architecture [18]. Compared to V2, Inception V3 reduces the number of

Table 1. Training statistics and testing performance

Feature	Training set (frames)	Testing set (videos)	Sensitivity (%)	Specificity (%)
B-line	16,300	212	28.0	93.0
Merged B-line	14,961	337	85.0	96.5
B-line (combined)	–	521	88.4	93.0
A-line	10,510	580	87.2	89.0
Pleural line	48,429	640	85.6	93.1
Pleural effusion	21,200	143	87.5	92.2
Consolidation	18,713	444	93.6	86.3
Pneumothorax	13,255*	35	93.0	93.0

*6,743 M-mode images with lung sliding, 6,512 M-mode images without lung sliding

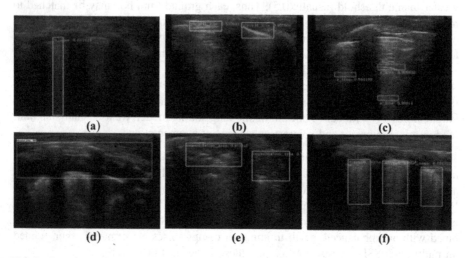

Fig. 4. Sample results for SSD detection models. Detected features are highlighted by bounding boxes and confidence scores. (A) B-line, (B) pleural line, (C) A-line, (D) pleural effusion, (E) consolidation, (F) merged B-line.

convolutions, limiting maximum filter size to 3 × 3, increases the depth of the network and uses an improved feature combination technique at each inception module. We initialized Inception V3 with pre-trained ImageNet weights and fine-tuned only the last two classification layers with virtual M-mode images. The network was trained for 10k iterations with batch size 100 and a constant learning rate of 0.001.

3 Results

We compare single class SSD performance with threshold-based detection methods [7, 20], which are effective only for pleural line and B-line features. The SSD framework is applicable to all lung ultrasound features and our SSD detection model detects pleural lines with 89% accuracy compared to 67% with threshold-based methods.

Our CNN models were evaluated against holdout test dataset acquired from two swine. Table 1 shows the final test results and Fig. 4 shows sample outputs for features other than lung sliding. The pleural effusion model detected effusion at all fluid volumes from 50 mL to 600 mL (300 mL shown). Pleural line was the most common lung feature, present in most ultrasound videos. Videos without pleural line were uncommon, making the specificity calculation unreliable. The absence of an intercostal space in a video was treated as a pleural line negative sample. Note that for consolidation, pleural effusion and merged B-lines, sensitivity and specificity metrics are defined on a per video basis, rather than per object.

The algorithm achieved at least 85% in sensitivity and specificity for all features, with the exception of B-line sensitivity. There exists a continuum of B-line density from single B-lines, to dense B-lines, to merged B-lines. We observed that in many cases, dense B-lines that were not detected by the B-line detection model were detected by the merged B-line model. We combined the B-line and merged B-line output with the idea that the distinction between these two classes may be poorly defined. The combined B-line model achieved 88.4% sensitivity and 93% specificity, which was significantly better than B-lines alone. The video-based pneumothorax model had the highest overall accuracy with 93% sensitivity and specificity.

4 Conclusions and Future Work

In summary, we demonstrated that a CNN-based computer vision algorithm can achieve a high level of concordance with an expert's observation of lung ultrasound images. Seven different lung features critical for diagnosing abnormal lung conditions were detected with greater than 85% accuracy. The algorithm in its current form would allow an ultrasound user with limited skill to identify the abnormal lung conditions outlined here. This work with swine models is an important step toward clinical trials with human patients, and an important proof of concept for the ability of computer vision algorithms to effect automated ultrasound image interpretation.

In the future, we will continue this work using clinical patient data. This will help validate the method's efficacy in humans while providing a sufficient diversity of patients and quantity of data to determine patient-level diagnostic accuracy. We are also working to implement this algorithm on tablets and smartphones. To help with runtime on mobile devices, we are streamlining the algorithm to combine the six parallel SSD models into a single multi-class model, while eliminating the need for coordinate transformations, which represents the bulk of the computational time during inference.

References

1. Litjens, G., et al.: A survey on deep learning in medical image analysis. Med. Image Anal. **42**, 60–88 (2017)
2. Testa, A., Soldati, G., Copetti, R., Giannuzzi, R., Portale, G., Gentiloni-Silveri, N.: Early recognition of the 2009 pandemic influenza A (H1N1) pneumonia by chest ultrasound. Crit. Care **16**(1), R30 (2011)
3. Parlamento, S., Copetti, R., Bartolomeo, S.D.: Evaluation of lung ultrasound for the diagnosis of pneumonia in the ED. Am. J. Emerg. **27**(4), 379–384 (2009)
4. Weitzel, W., Hamilton, J., Wang, X., Bull, J., Vollmer, A.: Quantitative lung ultrasound comet measurement: method and initial clinical results. Blood Purif. **39**, 37–44 (2015)
5. Anantrasirichai, N., Allinovi, M., Hayes, W., Achim, A.: Automatic B-line detection in paediatric lung ultrasound. In: 2016 IEEE International Ultrasonics Symposium (IUS), Tours, France (2016)
6. Moshavegh, R., et al.: Novel automatic detection of pleura and B-lines (comet-tail artifacts) on in vivo lung ultrasound scans. In: SPIE Medical Imaging 2016 (2016)
7. Fang, S., Wang, Y.R.B.: Automatic detection and evaluation of B-lines by lung ultrasound. NYU, New York City
8. Huang, Q., Zhang, F., Li, X.: Machine learning in ultrasound computer-aided diagnostic systems: a survey. BioMed Res. Int. (2018)
9. Jabbar, S., Day, C., Heinz, N., Chadwick, E.: Using Convolutional Neural Network for edge detection in musculoskeletal ultrasound images. In: International Joint Conference on Neural Networks, pp. 4619–4626 (2016)
10. Shin, J., Tajbakhsh, N., Hurst, R., Kendall, C., Liang, J.: Automating carotid intima-media thickness video interpretation with convolutional neural networks. In: Conference on Computer Vision and Pattern Recognition, Las Vegas, pp. 2526–2535 (2016)
11. Chen, H., et al.: Standard plane localization in fetal ultrasound via domain transferred deep neural networks. IEEE J. Biomed. Health Inform. **19**(5), 1627–1636 (2015)
12. Liu, W., et al.: SSD: Single Shot MultiBox Detector. In: Leibe, B., Matas, J., Sebe, N., Welling, M. (eds.) ECCV 2016. LNCS, vol. 9905, pp. 21–37. Springer, Cham (2016). https://doi.org/10.1007/978-3-319-46448-0_2
13. Volpicelli, G., et al.: International evidence-based recommendations for point-of-care lung ultrasound. Intensive Care Med. **38**(4), 577–591 (2012)
14. Girshick, R., Donahue, J., Darrell, T., Malik, J.: Rich feature hierarchies for accurate object detection and semantic segmentation. In: Proceedings of the IEEE Conference on Computer Vision and Pattern Recognition (CVPR), pp. 580–587 (2014)
15. Redmon, J., Divvala, S., Girshick, R., Farhadi, A.: You only look once: unified, real-time object detection. In: The IEEE Conference on Computer Vision and Pattern Recognition (CVPR), pp. 779–788 (2016)
16. Ren, S., He, K., Girshick, R., Sun, J.: Faster R-CNN: towards real-time object detection with region proposal networks. In: Advances in Neural Information Processing Systems (NIPS), pp. 91–99 (2015)
17. Huang, J., et al.: Speed/accuracy trade-offs for modern convolutional object detectors. In: The Conference on Computer Vision and Pattern Recognition (2017)
18. Szegedy, C., Vanhoucke, V., Loffe, S., Shlens, J., Wojna, Z.: Rethinking the inception architecture for computer vision. In: The Conference on Computer Vision and Pattern Recognition (2015)

19. Jia, D., Dong, W., Socher, R., Li, L.-J., Li, K., Fei-Fei, L.: ImageNet: a large-scale hierarchical image database. In: The Conference on Computer Vision and Pattern Recognition (2009)
20. Omar, Z., et al.: An explorative childhood pneumonia analysis based on ultrasonic imaging texture features. In: 11th International Symposium on Medical Information Processing and Analysis, vol. 9681 (2015)

Quantitative Echocardiography: Real-Time Quality Estimation and View Classification Implemented on a Mobile Android Device

Nathan Van Woudenberg[1], Zhibin Liao[1], Amir H. Abdi[1], Hani Girgis[2], Christina Luong[2], Hooman Vaseli[1], Delaram Behnami[1], Haotian Zhang[1], Kenneth Gin[2], Robert Rohling[1], Teresa Tsang[2(✉)], and Purang Abolmaesumi[1(✉)]

[1] University of British Columbia, Vancouver, BC, Canada
purang@ece.ubc.ca
[2] Vancouver General Hospital, Vancouver, BC, Canada
t.tsang@ubc.ca

Abstract. Accurate diagnosis in cardiac ultrasound requires high quality images, containing different specific features and structures depending on which of the 14 standard cardiac views the operator is attempting to acquire. Inexperienced operators can have a great deal of difficulty recognizing these features and thus can fail to capture diagnostically relevant heart cines. This project aims to mitigate this challenge by providing operators with real-time feedback in the form of view classification and quality estimation. Our system uses a frame grabber to capture the raw video output of the ultrasound machine, which is then fed into an Android mobile device, running a customized mobile implementation of the TensorFlow inference engine. By multi-threading four TensorFlow instances together, we are able to run the system at 30 Hz with a latency of under 0.4 s.

Keywords: Echocardiography · Deep learning · Mobile · Real time

1 Introduction

Ischaemic heart disease is the primary cause of death worldwide. Practicing effective preventative medicine of cardiovascular disease requires an imaging modality that can produce diagnostically relevant images, while at the same time being widely available, non-invasive, and cost-effective. Currently, the method that best fits these requirements is cardiac ultrasound (echocardiography, echo). Modern echo probes can be used to quickly and effectively evaluate the health of the patient's heart by assessing its internal structure and function [3]. The major

---

T. Tsang and P. Abolmaesumi—Joint senior authors.

© Springer Nature Switzerland AG 2018
D. Stoyanov et al. (Eds.): POCUS 2018/BIVPCS 2018/CuRIOUS 2018/CPM 2018,
LNCS 11042, pp. 74–81, 2018.
https://doi.org/10.1007/978-3-030-01045-4_9

caveat of this process is that the interpretation of these images is highly subject to the overall image quality of the captured cines, which, in turn, is dependent on both the patient's anatomy and the operator's skill. Poor quality echoes captured by inexperienced operators can jeopardize clinician interpretation and can thus adversely impact patient outcomes [8]. With the proliferation of portable ultrasound technology, more and more inexperienced users are picking up ultrasound probes and attempting to capture diagnostically relevant cardiac echoes without the required experience, skill or knowledge of heart anatomy.

In addition to the task of acquiring high quality images, ultrasound operators can also be expected to acquire up to 14 different cross-sectional 'views' of the heart, each with their own set of signature features. Some of these views are quite similar to an inexperience eye, and switching between them can require very precise adjustments of the probe's position and orientation. In point-of-care ultrasound (POCUS) environments, the four views most frequently acquired by clinicians are apical four-chamber (AP4), parasternal long axis (PLAX), parasternal short axis at the papillary muscle level (PSAX-PM), and subcostal four-chamber (SUBC4).

In this work, we attempt to reduce the adverse effect of inter-operator variability on the quality of the acquired cardiac echoes acquired. The system we developed attempts to do this by providing the user with real-time feedback of both view classification and image quality. This is done through the use of a deep learning neural network, capable of simultaneous 14-class view classification and a quality estimation score. Furthermore, we implemented the system in

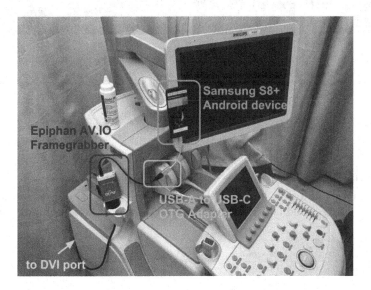

Fig. 1. The physical system setup. The frame grabber connects to the DVI output of the ultrasound machine. It is then connected to an OTG adapter and plugged directly into the Android's USB-C port.

the form of an Android application, and ran it on an off-the-shelf Samsung S8+ mobile phone, with the goal of making our system portable and cost effective. As shown in Fig. 1, the system receives its input directly from the DVI port of the ultrasound machine, using an Epiphan AV.IO frame grabber to capture and convert the raw video output to a serial data stream. The frame grabber output is then adapted from USB-A to USB-C with a standard On-The-Go (OTG) adapter, allowing us to pipe the ultrasound machine's video output directly into the Android device and through a neural network running on its CPU, using TensorFlow's Java inference interface. The classified view and its associated quality score are then displayed in the app's graphical user interface (GUI) as feedback to the operator. Figure 2 shows the feedback displayed in the GUI for four AP4 cines of differing quality levels. These four sample cines, from left to right, were scored by our expert echocardiographer as having image quality of 25%, 50%, 75%, and 100%, respectively.

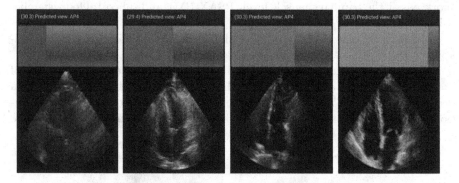

Fig. 2. The mobile application GUI showing the predicted view and quality for four different AP4 cines of increasing quality.

2   System Design

2.1   Deep Learning Design

A single deep learning network is used to learn the echo quality prediction and view classification for all 14 views. The model was trained on a dataset of over 16 K cines, distributed across the 14 views as shown in the following table:

Window	Apical				Parasternal						Subcostal			Suprasternal
view	AP2	AP3	AP4	AP5	PLAX	RVIF	$PSAX_A$	$PSAX_M$	$PSAX_{PM}$	$PSAX_{AP}$	SC4	SC5	IVC	SUPRA
# of cines	1,928	2,094	2,165	541	2,745	373	2,126	2,264	823	106	759	54	718	76

The network architecture can be seen in Fig. 3. The input to the network is a ten-frame tensor randomly extracted from an echo cine, and each frame is a

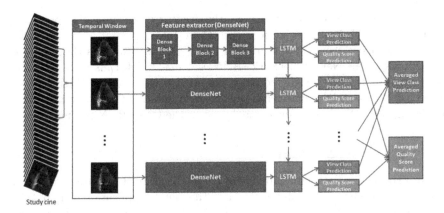

Fig. 3. The network architecture. Relevant features are extracted from the individual frames by the DenseNet blocks, which are then fed into the Long Short-Term Memory (LSTM) blocks to extract the temporal information across ten sequential echo cine frames.

120×120 pixel, gray-scale image. The network has four components, as shown in Fig. 3: (1) A seven-layer DenseNet [5] model that extracts per-frame features from the input; (2) an LSTM [4] layer with 128 units that captures the temporal dependencies from the generated DenseNet features, which produces another set of features, one for each frame; (3) a regression layer that produces the quality score from the output feature of the LSTM layer for each frame; and (4) a softmax classifier that predicts the content view from the LSTM features for each frame.

Our DenseNet model uses the following hyper-parameters. First, the DenseNet has one convolution layer with sixteen 3×3 filters, which turns the gray-scale (1-channel) input images to sixteen channels. Then, the DenseNet stacks three dense blocks, each followed by a dropout layer and an average-pooling layer with filter size of 2×2. Each dense block has exactly one dense-layer, which consists of a batch-normalized [6] convolution layer with six 3×3 filters and a Rectified Linear Unit (ReLU) [7] activation function. Finally, the per-frame quality scores and view predictions are averaged, respectively, to produce the final score and prediction for the ten-frame tensor.

2.2 Split Model

Initially, our system suffered from high latency due to the long inference times associated with running the entire network on an Android CPU. Since the network contains a ten-frame LSTM, we needed to buffer ten frames into a $120 \times 120 \times 10$ tensor, then run that tensor through both the Dense and LSTM layers of the network before getting any result. This produced a latency of up to 1.5 s, which users found frustrating and ultimately detrimental to the usefulness of the system.

In order to reduce the latency of the feedback, we split the previously described network into two sections: the Convolution Neural Network (CNN) section, which performs the feature extraction on each frame as they come in, and the Recurrent Neural Network (RNN) section, which runs on tensors now containing the features extracted from the previous ten frames. With the split model, we can essentially parallelize the feature extracting CNNs and the quality predicting RNN. See Fig. 6 for a visual view of the CNN/RNN timing.

2.3   Software Architecture

Figure 4 shows the data flow pipeline of the application. Input frames are captured by the frame grabber and are fed into the mobile application's Main Activity at a resolution of 640×480 at $30\,Hz$. We created a customized version of the UVCCamera library, openly licensed under Apache License, to access the frame grabber as an external web camera [2]. The application then crops the raw frames down to include only the ultrasound beam, the boundaries of which can be adjusted by the user. The cropped data is resized down to 120×120 to match the network's input dimensions. A copy of the full-resolution data is also saved for later expert evaluation. The resized data is then sent to an instance of TensorFlow Runner, a custom class responsible for preparing and running our data through the Android-Java implementation of the TensorFlow inference engine [1]. Here, we first perform a simple contrast enhancement step to mitigate the quality degradation introduced by the frame grabber. The frames are then sent to one of three identical Convolutional Neural Networks (CNN-1, CNN-2, or CNN-3). Each CNN runs in a separate thread in order to prevent lag during particularly long inference times. The extracted features are saved into a feature buffer which shared between all three threads. Once the shared feature buffer fills, the RNN thread is woken up and runs the buffered data through the LSTM portion of the network to produce the classification and quality predictions to be displayed in the GUI.

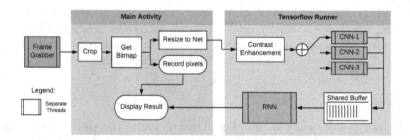

Fig. 4. Flow diagram of the software design.

3 Results

3.1 Classification

The training accuracy for the view classification was 92.35%, with a test accuracy of 86.21%. From the confusion matrix shown in Fig. 5, we can see that the majority of the classification error results from the parasternal short axis views, specifically $PSAX_M$, $PSAX_{PM}$, and $PSAX_{APIX}$. These 3 views are quite similar both visually and anatomically, and some of the cines in our training set contain frames from multiple PSAX views which may be confusing our classifier. The subcostal 5-chamber view also performed poorly, due to the small number of SC5 cines in our training set.

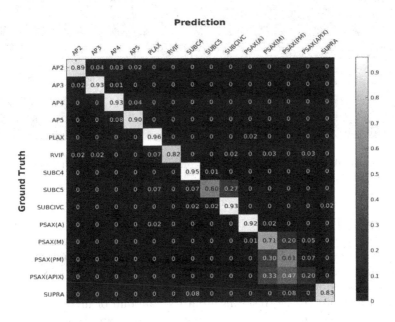

Fig. 5. The Confusion Matrix of the view classifier, showing all 14 heart views.

3.2 Timing

Since the system is required to run in real time on live data, the details regarding the timing are important to evaluating its performance. Figure 6 shows the timing profile of the three CNN threads, along with the single RNN thread, collected through Android Studio's CPU profiler tool. The three CNNs can be seen extracting features from ten consecutive input frames before waking the waiting RNN thread, which then runs the quality prediction on the buffered features extracted by the CNNs. The target frame rate for the system is set at 30 Hz, which can be inferred by the orange lines representing the arrival of

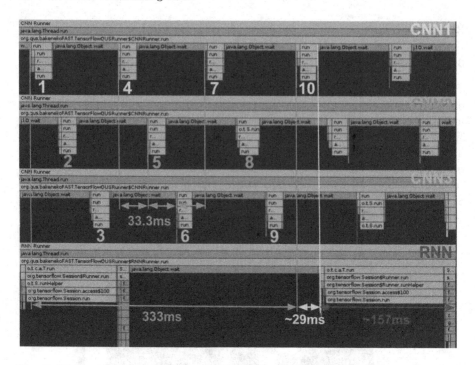

Fig. 6. Timing diagram of the three CNN and one RNN threads. The orange lines show the arrival of the input frames.

input frames. The mean CNN run-time (including feeding the input, running the network, and fetching the output) is 28.76 ms with an standard deviation of 16.42 ms. The mean run time of the RNN is 157.48 ms with a standard deviation of 21.85 ms. Therefore, the mean latency of the feedback is 352.58 ± 38.27 ms, when measured from the middle of the ten-frame sequence.

In order to prevent lag resulting from the build-up of unprocessed frames, the CNNs and RNN need to finish running before they are requested to process the next batch of data. To accomplish this reliably, all the per-frame processing must complete within $T_{max,CNN}$, calculated as follows:

$$T_{max,CNN} = (\# \text{ of CNNs}) \times \frac{1}{\text{FPS}} = \frac{3}{30} = 100 \; ms \qquad (1)$$

while the RNN needs to complete its processing before the features from the next ten frames are extracted:

$$T_{max,RNN} = (\text{buffer length}) \times \frac{1}{\text{FPS}} = \frac{10}{30} = 333.33 \, \text{ms} \qquad (2)$$

With the chosen three-CNN-one-RNN configuration, the application required the fewest number of threads while still providing enough tolerance to avoid frame build-up.

4 Discussion

In this paper, we present a system that provides ultrasound operators with real-time feedback about the heart echoes being captured, in the form of view classification and image quality estimation. The system is implemented in an Android application on an off-the-shelf Samsung S8+ and can be connected to any ultrasound machine with a DVI output port. In order to reduce the latency of the system, the neural network is split into two sections: the CNN and the RNN, allowing us to parallelize their execution. With the split model, the system is able to operate at 30 frames per second, while providing feedback with a mean latency of 352.91 ± 38.27 ms.

The next step of this project is to validate the system in a clinical setting. Our group is currently running a study at Vancouver General Hospital, in which we ask subjects to acquire cines of the four POCUS views once with and once without displaying the quality and view feedback in the app. The two datasets will be scored by expert echocardiographers and then compared in order to quantify the accuracy and utility of the system. We also plan to migrate the backend to TensorFlow Lite, a lightweight implementation of the inference engine, which will allow us to leverage the hardware acceleration available on modern Android devices to help us further reduce the system's latency.

Acknowledgements. The authors wish to thank the Natural Sciences and Engineering Research Council of Canada (NSERC) and the Canadian Institutes for Health Research (CIHR) for funding this project. We would like to also thank Dale Hawley from the Vancouver Coastal Health Information Technology for providing us access to the echo data during the development of this project.

References

1. Tensorflow android camera demo. https://github.com/tensorflow/tensorflow/tree/master/tensorflow/examples/android. Accessed 4 Feb 2018
2. Uvccamera. https://github.com/saki4510t/UVCCamera. Accessed 16 Dec 2017
3. Ciampi, Q., Pratali, L., Citro, R., Piacenti, M., Villari, B., Picano, E.: Identification of responders to cardiac resynchronization therapy by contractile reserve during stress echocardiography. Eur. J. Heart Failure **11**(5), 489–496 (2009)
4. Hochreiter, S., Schmidhuber, J.: Long short-term memory. Neural Comput. **9**(8), 1735–1780 (1997)
5. Huang, G., Liu, Z., Weinberger, K.Q., van der Maaten, L.: Densely connected convolutional networks. In: IEEE CVPR, vol. 1–2, p. 3 (2017)
6. Ioffe, S., Szegedy, C.: Batch normalization: accelerating deep network training by reducing internal covariate shift. In: Proceedings of the 32nd International Conference on Machine Learning, ICML 2015, pp. 448–456. JMLR (2015)
7. Nair, V., Hinton, G.E.: Rectified linear units improve restricted Boltzmann machines. In: Proceedings of the 27th International Conference on Machine Learning (ICML-2010), pp. 807–814 (2010)
8. Tighe, D.A., et al.: Influence of image quality on the accuracy of real time three-dimensional echocardiography to measure left ventricular volumes in unselected patients: a comparison with gated-spect imaging. Echocardiography **24**(10), 1073–1080 (2007)

Single-Element Needle-Based Ultrasound Imaging of the Spine: An *In Vivo* Feasibility Study

Haichong K. Zhang, Younsu Kim, Abhay Moghekar[(✉)], Nicholas J. Durr, and Emad M. Boctor[(✉)]

Johns Hopkins University, Baltimore, MD 21218, USA
{hzhang61,ykim99,ndurr}@jhu.edu, {am,eboctor1}@jhmi.edu

Abstract. Spinal interventional procedures, such as lumbar puncture, require insertion of an epidural needle through the spine without touching the surrounding bone structures. To minimize the number of insertion trials and navigate to a desired target, an image-guidance technique is necessary. We developed a single-element needle-based ultrasound system that is composed of a needle-shaped ultrasound transducer that reconstructs B-mode images from lateral movement with synthetic aperture focusing. The objective of this study is to test the feasibility of needle-based single-element ultrasound imaging on spine *in vivo*. Experimental validation was performed on a metal wire phantom, *ex vivo* porcine bone in both water tank and porcine tissue, and spine on living swine model. The needle-based ultrasound system could visualize the structure, although reverberation and multiple reflections associated with the needle shaft were observed. These results show the potential of the system to be used for *in vivo* environment.

Keywords: Needle-based ultrasound · Synthetic aperture focusing
Spinal intervention · Single-element ultrasound imaging

1 Introduction

Lumbar puncture (LP) is an interventional procedure for collecting cerebrospinal fluid (CSF), which is used to diagnose central nervous system disorders such as encephalitis or meningitis [1]. LP requires inserting a needle into the lower lumbar intervertebral space, and conventional LP is mostly performed without image assistance or guidance. This often results in misdiagnosis or damage to surrounding neurovascular structures [2–6]. Obese patients with thick adipose tissue layers further complicate the procedure, and consequently the rate of overall complications doubles compared to non-obese patients [7,8]. Many image-guided solutions have been proposed to resolve this challenge. A typical approach

---

H. K. Zhang and Y. Kim—Equal contribution.

D. Stoyanov et al. (Eds.): POCUS 2018/BIVPCS 2018/CuRIOUS 2018/CPM 2018,
LNCS 11042, pp. 82–89, 2018.
https://doi.org/10.1007/978-3-030-01045-4_10

is to project needle position into external medical imaging modalities such as ultrasound or CT [9–11]. However, this approach not only increases the cost by introducing bulky systems, but also has a limited tracking accuracy depending on the registration performance. Moreover, image quality of topical ultrasound degrades with obese patients, where the technology is most-needed. A low-cost and registration-free guidance system that provides an image through a needle that can be navigated through soft tissues could improve deep needle procedures such as challenging LPs.

Here, we propose a simple and direct needle insertion platform, enabling image formation from sweeping a needle with single element ultrasound transducer at its tip. This needle-embedded ultrasound transducer can not only provide one-dimensional depth information as Chiang et al. reported [12,13], but also visually locate the structures by combining transducer location tracking and a synthetic aperture focusing algorithm [14,15]. This system can minimize the hardware cost for production due to its simplicity, and more importantly does not require registration process as the needle and ultrasound images are co-registered by nature. In the prior study, we built a proto-type system which consists of a needle-shape transducer and a mounting holster that tracks the rotational position of the needle [16,17]. While the developed system could image wire and spine phantom inside the water tank, the remaining question was that if the system can provide sufficient contrast from a spine under practical environments, where the spine is covered by muscle and fat tissue layers. Therefore, this paper focuses on the validation of the technique with the presence of realistic tissue layers through both *ex vivo* and *in vivo* experiments.

2   Materials and Methods

2.1   Needle-Based Ultrasound Imaging and Synthetic Aperture Focusing

The proposed needle-based ultrasound imaging system is a needle-shaped device that functions as an ultrasound transducer. This transducer can transmit and receive ultrasound signals, and collects A-line data. By tracking the position of the needle while applying the motion, a virtual array is formed to build a B-mode image [18]. From the image, the operator can identify the position and angle of needle insertion. Synthetic aperture focusing is the reconstruction step to synthesize coherent sub-aperture information at each position of the needle and to form a final image with higher resolution and contrast. In this paper, the translational motion was applied using a translation stage.

2.2   Experiment Setup

As the imaging system, a needle-shaped ultrasound transducer (ndtXducer, USA) that includes the PZT-5H element on the tip was used. The diameter of the element was 1 mm, and its center frequency is 2.17 MHz with a -6db bandwidth of 0.32 MHz. The electrodes of the element are connected to a coaxial cable with a BNC connector so that the needle could be connected to sampling devices. For ultrasound pulse generation and A-line ultrasound signal sampling, US-WAVE (Lecouer, France) was connected to the element electrodes with a 100 Ω input impedance. The needle was fixed on a translation stage, and we moved it in 0.5 mm steps to form a virtual linear array.

The developed system was tested with a metal rod phantom as well as *ex vivo* and *in vivo* porcine spine. For the *ex vivo* study, the porcine spine was placed inside the water tank to confirm the contrast from the bone without the tissue layer first. Then, a porcine muscle tissue layer with 2–3 cm thickness was placed on the top of spine and imaged. The image quality of phantom and *ex vivo* targets was quantified using the contrast-to-noise ratio (CNR) to evaluate the effect of synthetic aperture focusing [18]. Finally, the spine of a Yorkshire pig was imaged for *in vivo* validation, where the dorsal part of the pig was faced top, and the imaging system was fixed on the translation stage and placed above skin surface. Ultrasound gel and water covered by plastic frame and plastic wrap were used for acoustic coupling. The pig was anesthetized, and minimal respiratory motion was maintained during the imaging sessions (Fig. 1).

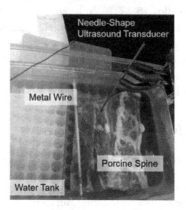

Fig. 1. Experimental setup of phantom and *ex vivo* experiments. The needle-shape ultrasound transducer is held by a gripper which is connected to a translation stage.

3   Results

3.1   Phantom Study

Figure 2 shows the imaging result of the metal rod phantom. Without synthetic aperture focusing, the metal rod structure was defocused because there is no acoustic focus embedded in the single element transducer (CNR: 2.61). With the synthetic aperture focusing, the metal rod shape appears as its original shape and size (CNR: 5.45) although reverberation and multi-reflections are observed beyond the metal rod due to the single-element needle structure. The speed-of-sound was set to 1490 m/s, the aperture size of 40 mm was used in beamforming.

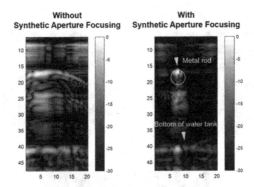

Fig. 2. The needle-based ultrasound images of the metal rod with and without synthetic aperture focusing. The numerical scale is mm.

3.2   *Ex Vivo* Demonstration

We tested the visibility of *ex vivo* porcine spine under two conditions. In the first condition, we placed porcine spine bones surrounded by thin muscle tissue at the bottom of a water tank. A clinical ultrasound scanner (SonixTouch, Ultrasonix, Canada) with a convex probe (C5-2, Ultrasonix, Canada) was used to confirm the bone structure for reference. We collected A-line data at 80 positions by moving in 0.5 mm steps in the sagittal plane direction. In Fig. 3, two images are shown for comparison: an image built without synthetic aperture focusing, and the other image with synthetic aperture focusing, where the aperture size of 40 mm was used. Although a bone structure located at the left side of the images was depicted in both images, the other bone located at the right side of the images is clearly visible only in the image with synthetic aperture focusing. The CNR improvement was from 2.15 to 7.13, corresponding to before and after synthetic aperture focusing.

In the second condition, we performed spine bone imaging through porcine muscle tissue to observe the tolerance to a more challenging environment. We stacked a porcine muscle layer on top of the spine bone. The received echo signals were attenuated more compared to the previous *ex vivo* experiment in the water tank. Two bone structures were confirmed in the synthetic aperture focusing image (CNR: 2.65) while these structures were barely visible before applying the synthetic aperture focusing (CNR: 1.20) (Fig. 4).

3.3   *In Vivo* Demonstration

A spine of Yorkshire pig was imaged for *in vivo* validation. We scanned the porcine spine from both sagittal and transverse planes. In both cases, the imaging needle was translated for 40 mm corresponding to 80 positions. We used a commercially available convex probe (C3, Clarius, Canada) for reference. To minimize the effect of motion artifact, the aperture size of 20 mm was used in beamforming. Figures 5 and 6 show the results. For the sagittal view, two spinous

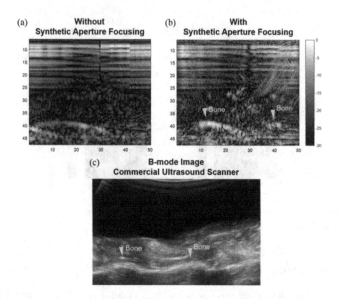

Fig. 3. The needle-based ultrasound images of *ex vivo* porcine spine placed inside the water tank. (a) Before and (b) after applying synthetic aperture focusing. The numerical scale is mm. (c) The reference image taken at the similar region using a commercial ultrasound scanner.

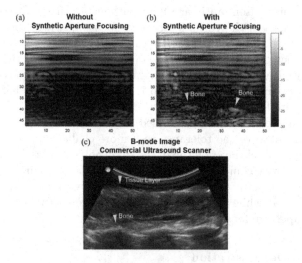

Fig. 4. The needle-based ultrasound images of *ex vivo* porcine spine placed under the porcine tissue. (a) Before and (b) after applying synthetic aperture focusing. The numerical scale is mm. (c) The reference image taken at the similar region using a commercial ultrasound scanner.

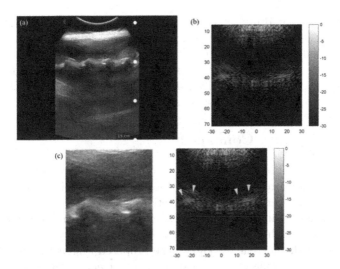

Fig. 5. Experimental results of *in vivo* porcine spine images in the sagittal plane. (a) The reference image taken using a commercial ultrasound scanner, and (b) the needle-based ultrasound image. The numerical scale is mm. (c) The comparison of the highlighted region of (a) (left) and (b) (right). The yellow arrow indicates the bone structure. (Color figure online)

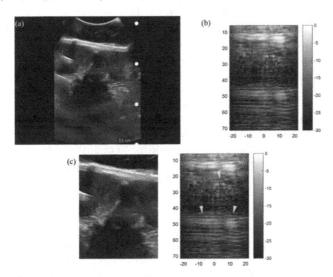

Fig. 6. Experimental results of *in vivo* porcine spine images in the transverse plane. (a) The reference image taken using a commercial ultrasound scanner, and (b) the needle-based ultrasound image. The numerical scale is mm. (c) The comparison of the highlighted region of (a) (left) and (b) (right). The yellow arrow indicates the bone structure. (Color figure online)

processes were captured in the needle-based ultrasound image, and the position of these processes matched with that in the reference image. For the transverse view, it was challenging to confirm the same structure visible in the reference image, but the signal from the processes and facet could be seen in the synthetic aperture focusing image. Nonetheless, the imaging system suffers from the noises caused by respiratory motion, ultrasound reverberations and multi-reflections.

4   Discussion and Conclusion

The current standard of care for LP introduces a wide range of iatrogenic complications and places a heavy financial burden on the patient, physician, and healthcare system overall. Our cost-effective single-needle ultrasound system would lead to fewer unnecessary and expensive consequent procedures. Point of care ultrasound technologies need to provide a solution that is built around efficiency within the current workflow. The proposed system accomplishes this by implementing an imaging modality into the current needle itself, providing those important advantages. With addition of the imaging modality, physicians can be trained for LP in a shorter time, without the hassle of keeping track of a separate imaging probe.

In this work, we showed the feasibility of the proposed system under *in vivo* environment and the potential for clinical translation. However, the reconstructed images suffer from artifacts and noises caused by the current needle structure and the sampling device. The image quality can be enhanced by improving the needle fabrication and signal sampling and processing method.

Acknowledgements. The authors would like to acknowledge Mateo Paredes, Karun Kannan, Shayan Roychoudhury for their contributions to the project in a variety of capacities. Financial supports were provided by Johns Hopkins University internal funds, NIH Grant No. R21CA202199, and NIGMS-/NIBIB-NIH Grant No. R01EB021396, NSF SCH:CAREER Grant No. 1653322, and CDMRP PCRP No. W81XWH1810188. The authors also acknowledge VentureWell, the Coulter Translational Foundation, and the Maryland Innovation Initiative, and the Steven & Alexandra Cohen Foundation for their support throughout this project.

References

1. Koster-Rasmussen, R., Korshin, A., Meyer, C.N.: Antibiotic treatment delay and outcome in acute bacterial meningitis. J. Infect. **57**(6), 449–454 (2008)
2. Armon, C., Evans, R.W.: Addendum to assessment: prevention of post-lumbar puncture headaches. Neurology **65**, 510–512 (2005)
3. American Society for Healthcare Risk Management, "Risk Management Handbook for Health Care Organizations", vol. 5. Jossey-Bass (2009)
4. Edwards, C., Leira, E.C., Gonzalez-Alegre, P.: Residency training: a failed lumbar puncture is more about obesity than lack of ability. Neurology **84**(10), e69–72 (2015)
5. Shah, K.H., Richard, K.M.: Incidence of traumatic lumbar puncture. Acad. Emerg. Med. **10**(2), 151–4 (2003)

6. Ahmed, S.V., Jayawarna, C., Jude, E.: Post lumbar puncture headache: diagnosis and management. Postgrad. Med. J. **82**(273), 713–716 (2006)
7. Shaikh, F., et al.: Ultrasound imaging for lumbar punctures and epidural catheterisations: systematic review and meta-analysis. BMJ **346**, f1720 (2013)
8. Brook, A.D., Burns, J., Dauer, E., Schoendfeld, A.H., Miller, T.S.: Comparison of CT and fluoroscopic guidance for lumbar puncture in an obese population with prior failed unguided attempt. J. NeuroInterventional Surg. **6**, 323–327 (2014)
9. Tamas, U., et al.: Spinal needle navigation by tracked ultrasound snapshots. IEEE Trans. Biomed. Eng. **59**(10), 2766–72 (2012)
10. Chen, E.C.S., Mousavi, P., Gill, S., Fichtinger, G., Abolmaesumi, P.: Ultrasound guided spine needle insertion. Proc. SPIE **7625**, 762538 (2010)
11. Najafi, M., Abolmaesumi, P., Rohling, R.: Single-camera closed-form real-time needle tracking for ultrasound-guided needle insertion. Ultrasound Med. Biol. **41**(10), 2663–2676 (2015)
12. Chiang, H.K.: Eyes in the needle, novel epidural needle with embedded high-frequency ultrasound transducer-epidural access in porcine model. J. Am. Soc. Anesthesiologists **114**(6), 1320–1324 (2011)
13. Lee, P.-Y., Huang, C.-C., Chiang, H.K.: Implementation of a novel high frequency ultrasound device for guiding epidural anesthesia-in vivo animal study. In: Proceedings of IEEE (2013)
14. Jensen, J.A., Nikolov, S.I., Gammelmark, K.L., Pedersen, M.H.: Synthetic aperture ultrasound imaging. Ultrasonics **44**(22), e5–e15 (2006)
15. Zhang, H.K., Cheng, A., Bottenus, N., Guo, X., Trahey, G.E., Boctor, E.M.: Synthetic Tracked Aperture Ultrasound (STRATUS) imaging: design, simulation, and experimental evaluation. J. Med. Imaging **3**(2), 027001 (2016)
16. Zhang, H.K., Kim, Y.: Toward dynamic lumbar puncture guidance using needle-based single-element ultrasound imaging. J. Med. Imaging **5**(2), 021224 (2018)
17. Zhang, H.K., Lin, M., Kim, Y., et al.: Toward dynamic lumbar punctures guidance based on single element synthetic tracked aperture ultrasound imaging. In: Proceedings of SPIE, vol. 10135, p. 101350J (2017)
18. Üstüner, K.F., Holley, G.L.: Ultrasound imaging system performance assessment. In: Presented at the 2003 American Association of Physicists in Medicine Annual Meeting, San Diego, CA (2003)

International Workshop
on Bio-Imaging and Visualization
for Patient-Customized Simulations,
BIVPCS 2018

A Novel Interventional Guidance Framework for Transseptal Puncture in Left Atrial Interventions

Pedro Morais[1,2,3,4]($\boxtimes$), João L. Vilaça[3,4,5], Sandro Queirós[2,3,4,6],
Pedro L. Rodrigues[3,4], João Manuel R. S. Tavares[1], and Jan D'hooge[2]

[1] Instituto de Ciência e Inovação em Engenharia Mecânica e Engenharia Industrial, Departamento de Engenharia Mecânica, Faculdade de Engenharia, Universidade do Porto, Porto, Portugal
pedromorais@med.uminho.pt
[2] Lab on Cardiovascular Imaging and Dynamics, Department of Cardiovascular Sciences, KULeuven - University of Leuven, Leuven, Belgium
[3] Life and Health Sciences Research Institute (ICVS), School of Medicine, University of Minho, Braga, Portugal
[4] ICVS/3B's-PT, Government Associate Laboratory, Braga, Guimarães, Portugal
[5] 2Ai-Technology School, Polytechnic Institute of Cávado and Ave, Barcelos, Portugal
[6] Algoritmi Center, School of Engineering, University of Minho, Guimarães, Portugal

Abstract. Access to the left atrium is required for several percutaneous cardiac interventions. In these procedures, the inter-atrial septal wall is punctured using a catheter inserted in the right atrium under image guidance. Although this approach (transseptal puncture - TSP) is performed daily, complications are common. In this work, we present a novel concept for the development of an interventional guidance framework for TSP. The pre-procedural planning stage is fused with 3D intra-procedural images (echocardiography) using manually defined landmarks, transferring the relevant anatomical landmarks to the interventional space and enhancing the echocardiographic images. In addition, electromagnetic sensors are attached to the surgical instruments, tracking and including them in the enhanced intra-procedural world. Two atrial phantom models were used to evaluate this framework. To assess its accuracy, a metallic landmark was positioned in the punctured location and compared with the ideal one. The intervention was possible in both models, but in one case positioning of the landmark failed. An error of approximately of 6 mm was registered for the successful case. Technical characteristics of the framework showed an acceptable performance (frame rate ~ 5 frames/s). This study presented a proof-of-concept for an interventional guidance framework for TSP. However, a more automated solution and further studies are required.

Keywords: Image-guided cardiac interventions · Transseptal puncture
Image fusion · Echocardiography
Integrated interventional guidance framework

© Springer Nature Switzerland AG 2018
D. Stoyanov et al. (Eds.): POCUS 2018/BIVPCS 2018/CuRIOUS 2018/CPM 2018,
LNCS 11042, pp. 93–101, 2018.
https://doi.org/10.1007/978-3-030-01045-4_11

1 Introduction

Access to the left atrium (LA) is mandatory in multiple minimally invasive cardiac interventions, such as left atrial appendage closure, atrial fibrillation ablation, mitral valve replacement, among others [1, 2]. Since no direct percutaneous access route to LA is available, a transseptal via is typically used. For that, a medical technique termed transseptal puncture (TSP) is applied, where a catheter is inserted via the femoral vein until the right atrium (RA), through which a needle is moved forward to puncture the inter-atrial septal (IAS) wall (using its thinnest region, the fossa ovalis - FO) and gain access to the LA body [2]. This procedure is guided using medical images, namely fluoroscopy and echocardiography (mainly transesophageal echocardiography - TEE) [1]. Nevertheless, the success of the intervention is still highly dependent on the operator's expertise, which is sub-optimal. Indeed, when puncturing the IAS, not only the FO needs to be identified, but also the target location at the left heart and the catheter dexterity at this region must be taken into consideration, hampering the identification of the optimal puncture location [1].

To improve the TSP intervention, different technological innovations were presented during the last years. Three major development fields can be considered, namely: surgical tools, pre-procedural planning techniques and guidance approaches [1]. A high number of researchers focused on the former, presenting novel radio-frequency/electrocautery needles (instead of the traditional mechanical ones), which proved their clear advantages for abnormal situations [2]. Regarding the planning techniques, a small number of studies were presented, focusing on biomechanical simulation of the intervention [3] or automated identification of relevant landmarks (e.g. fossa ovalis position) [4], making the planning stage faster and more reproducible. Regarding the intraoperative guidance, several researchers explored the potential use of novel imaging modalities (beyond the traditional ones, magnetic resonance imaging – MRI, and intracardiac echocardiography) for TSP [1]. Moreover, electroanatomical mapping solutions or even electromagnetic guidance solutions were also described [1]. More recently, some researchers presented image-fusion strategies [6–8], where the bidimensional and low contrast fluoroscopic image is fused with 3D anatomical detailed models (extracted from echocardiography or computed tomography - CT), showing clear advantages for TSP with inferior procedural time and higher success rate in difficult cases. Nevertheless, although such image fusion solutions showed high potential to ease the intervention [6–8], most of them fuse intra-procedural images only (not allowing the inclusion of pre-procedural planning information) or were not validated for TSP.

In this study, we present a novel concept for the development of an integrated interventional guidance framework to assist the physician in successfully performing TSP intervention.

2   Methods

The proposed interventional framework is divided into (Fig. 1): (1) the pre-procedural and (2) the intra-procedural stages. During the first stage, identification or delineation (step A) of relevant cardiac chambers in a highly-detailed image (CT) is performed. Then, based on the estimated contours, the full extent of the FO is estimated and the optimal puncture location is defined by the expert (step B). The entire planning information is then transferred to the intra-procedural world (step C), by fusing intra- and pre-procedural data (e.g. contours or landmarks). Note that intra-procedural data is extracted from echocardiographic images only (in this initial setup, transthoracic echocardiography – TTE – was used). Finally, to also include the surgical instruments into this augmented environment, a tracking strategy is applied using external electromagnetic sensors (step D). An initial calibration between the TTE image world and the electromagnetic sensors was required (step E). By combining all these elements (step F), a radiation-free interventional framework with enhanced anatomical information (from the planning stage) is achieved.

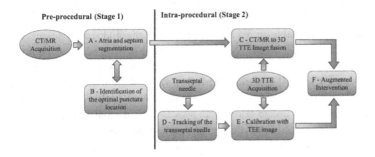

Fig. 1. Blocks diagram of the proposed concept.

2.1   Interventional Framework

The interventional framework was implemented in C++ and it exploits the potentialities of the VTK (Visualization Toolkit) library [11] for the visualization of images/surfaces and even 3D rendering (using OpenGL). The framework has 4 independent views (see Fig. 2), allowing the visualization of the pre- and intra-procedural data through 2D views or 3D renderings. The current version implements the intra-procedural guidance stage only, presenting import functions to include the pre-procedural planning data. Moreover, specific libraries to receive, in real-time, 3D TTE images (from a commercially available ultrasound – US - machine) and the 3D position of the different instruments were used.

As such, the different steps of the described concept were implemented as (Fig. 2):

Step A: A manual delineation of the LA and RA was performed using the Medical Imaging Interaction Toolkit (MITK) software. In detail, multiple 2D slices were delineated and then interpolated into a 3D surface. Each surface was independently delineated and saved in stl (stereolitrography) format.

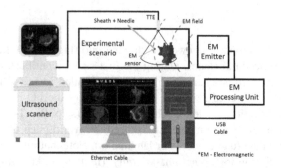

Fig. 2. Overview of the developed interventional setup.

Step B: Based on the 3D contours from (A), the FO was manually identified. For that, we detected the thinnest region, as described in [4]. Then, the optimal puncture location was marked and saved in stl format.

Step C: Both pre-procedural (CT) and intra-procedural (TTE) images were uploaded and streamed in the described framework (Fig. 2), respectively. The CT image is uploaded using the DICOM (Digital Imaging and Communications in Medicine) read function currently available in VTK. In opposition, the TTE images were acquired in real-time with a Vivid E95 (GE Vingmed, Horten, Norway) scanner, equipped with a 4 V-D transducer and streamed using a proprietary software. Regarding the image-fusion between CT and TTE worlds, the following strategy was applied. By visualizing both images in parallel, a set of landmarks were manually defined in both images, being later used to fuse both image coordinate space. The optimal transformation between CT-TTE worlds was computed through a least-square strategy. After estimating the optimal transformation, the surfaces generated throughout steps A and B are imported and automatically superimposed on the intra-procedural image, enhancing the relevant anatomical landmarks.

Step D: A small electromagnetic (EM) sensor (EM, Fig. 2) with 6 degrees of freedom (DOF), Aurora 6DOF Flex Tube, Type 2 (Aurora, Northern Digital, Waterloo, Ontario), was attached to the tip of the transseptal sheath.

Step E: A fixed calibration was made to combine the electromagnetic and TTE worlds. In this sense, a set of positions were identified in the TTE image. Then, the same spatial positions were physically achieved by the EM sensor, and the final optimal transformation was obtained by applying a least-square fitting between all positions. By applying this spatial transformation, a unique scenario combining the enhanced intra-procedural image with the needle position was obtained, allowing the correct guidance of the surgical tool until the optimal puncture location. Inside the proposed guidance framework, the needle position was represented as a red dot.

3   Experiments

Description: In this version, two patient-specific mock models of the atria were used (Fig. 3). Both static models were constructed using the strategy described in [10].

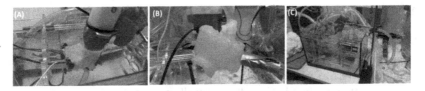

Fig. 3. Experimental validation scenario.

Implementation Details: Since mock models were used, the TTE probe was kept fixed (Fig. 3). Before executing the calibration, one operator selected the optimal field of the view (FOV) of the model. Regarding the identification of relevant landmarks (step C and E), Fig. 4 presents an overview of the target positions.

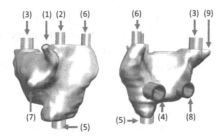

Fig. 4. Relevant landmark positions for step C and E.

Evaluation: One operator applied the described pipeline in each phantom model and then performed a TSP. To evaluate the error between the selected location and the puncture position, a metallic landmark was later inserted to mark the punctured site. Later, a CT acquisition of the model plus the landmark was acquired. This post-interventional CT was segmented and the obtained surfaces were aligned with the planning surfaces using an iterative closest point algorithm. Finally, the frame rate achieved by the framework for the streaming of US data was also evaluated. All results were computed using a personal laptop with Intel (R) i7 CPU at 2.8 GHz and 16 GB of RAM. An integrated graphics card Nvidia Quadro K2100 was used.

4   Results

The TSP was possible in both cases. Overall, guidance with this setup was considered challenging, due to limited information about the TSP needle position. In one phantom model, an error of approximately 6 mm was found between the selected position and the metallic landmark. For the second model, it was not possible to insert the metallic landmark. Regarding the technical characteristics, a frame rate of approximately 5 frames/s was achieved. The technical calibration took ~ 60 min. The planning stage required ~ 30 min.

5 Discussion

In this study, a novel interventional framework for TSP is described. It uses the potentialities of the intra-procedural volumetric US image to create an integrated interventional scenario where both pre-planning, intra-procedural data, and surgical instrument position are fused. Thus, the not well contrasted and noisy TTE image is enhanced by superimposing virtual anatomical surfaces. Moreover, the optimal puncture location can also be visualized, potentially increasing the safety of the intervention. In opposition to other studies [11], the current concept allows the inclusion of pre-procedural planning information in the interventional world. Indeed, recent solutions, such as the EchoNavigator (Philips Inc., Netherlands), [12] proved its added-value for TSP intervention, by adding anatomical information (US images) to the fluoroscopy. Nevertheless, although this solution allows the inclusion of specific landmarks in the interventional image, one is not able to embed pre-procedural planning information in the intra-procedural world [12]. In a different way, CT-fluoroscopy fusion approach was also described and validated for TSP [7], allowing the usage of pre-procedural data into the interventional scenario. However, since the US image is not integrated, relevant online anatomical details are lost or ultimately require an independent US scanner during the intervention.

This framework has as a key novelty the direct usage of 3D US data (by streaming it) to fuse intra-procedural data with pre-procedural one. In fact, previous works focused on similar methodologies for different scenarios. Nevertheless, 2D US data was mainly streamed, requiring complex calibration scenarios to perform 2D-3D alignment [11, 14]. Although such approaches have shown interesting results in nearly static structures/organs [12], its application in cardiac interventions is limited. As such, by capturing the entire 3D volume, 2D-3D alignment/reconstruction steps are removed, potentially improving the performance and accuracy of image-fusion algorithms. However, the described pipeline is only an initial proof-of-concept and it still presents some drawbacks, namely manual interaction is mandatory in all stages, making the configuration of the setup extremely time-consuming. Recently, our team has presented different methodologies to automate this framework: (1) automatic segmentation of the atrial region in CT [4, 15]; (2) automatic identification of the FO in CT [4]; and (3) automatic segmentation of the LA [16]. As such, the entire planning can be performed quickly (2–3 min, [4]) and the fusion stage can be quickly performed by aligning the segmented models. Although the current automated modules are not integrated into this framework, such options are expected in a future release. Regarding the tracking of the different surgical tools, fixed calibration setups can be used [11], making its calibration fast. Nevertheless, to improve the guidance of the surgical tools and the identification of the optimal puncture route, two modifications should be performed to the current setup: (i) multiple sensors should be embedded along the instrument, providing a virtual representation of the entire instrument's shape inside the body, and (ii) an enhanced representation of the optimal puncture route can potentiate the guidance stage and facilitate the identification of the puncture location. Finally, regarding the frame rate, an acceptable performance (5 frames/s) was achieved by this framework.

The obtained results showed that accurate evaluation of the proposed framework was not possible. First, a small number of phantom models were used. Second, the strategy applied to mark the punctured location proved to be sub-optimal. Due to the small entry points of the phantom model, visual identification punctured location was challenging, hampering the insertion of the metallic landmark. Third, quantification of the framework's accuracy through the described approach (i.e. aligning post-interventional data with pre-interventional one) is sensitive to small alignment errors. In this sense and to improve the described experiment, a novel scenario is required with the following features: (1) a large number of phantom models with different anatomies are required; (2) inclusion of radiopaque materials to easily allow an accurate alignment between the pre- and pos- interventional surfaces; and (3) instead of using metallic landmarks, the TSP needle should be kept at the punctured location. Finally, since the traditional intervention is widely dependent of the fluoroscopy, further studies to evaluate the feasibility of this potential radiation-free framework and even to evaluate the required learning curve are mandatory to validate it. Regarding the study limitations, we would like to emphasize that: (1) static phantom models were used; (2) instead of a TEE probe, a TTE one was used; and (3) the US probe was kept fixed throughout the intervention. To overcome these limitations, dynamic phantom setups, as described in [10], should be used, and an electromagnetic sensor should be attached to the ultrasound probe (as described in [14]), spatially relating the ultrasound FOV with the probe position and allowing its free manipulation throughout the intervention. As a final remark, although this study was performed with a TTE transducer (since it was simple to be fixated), the TEE one can also be used without any modification of the current setup.

6   Conclusion

The described concept for the development of an interventional guidance framework showed its initial potential usefulness for the identification of the optimal puncture location and to guide the TSP intervention. Nevertheless, the current version requires manual interaction in all stages, making the configuration setup extremely time-consuming and difficult to be performed. Further studies and a different experimental setup are required to accurately validate the proposed framework.

Acknowledgments. The authors acknowledge Fundação para a Ciência e a Tecnologia (FCT), in Portugal, and the European Social Found, European Union, for funding support through the "Programa Operacional Capital Humano" (POCH) in the scope of the PhD grants SFRH/BD/95438/2013 (P. Morais) and SFRH/BD/93443/2013 (S. Queirós).

This work was funded by projects NORTE-01-0145-FEDER-000013, NORTE-01-0145-FEDER-000022 and NORTE-01-0145-FEDER-024300, supported by Northern Portugal Regional Operational Programme (Norte2020), under the Portugal 2020 Partnership Agreement, through the European Regional Development Fund (FEDER), and has also been funded by FEDER funds, through Competitiveness Factors Operational Programme (COMPETE), and by national funds, through the FCT, under the scope of the project POCI-01-0145-FEDER-007038.

The authors would like to acknowledge Walter Coudyzer and Steven Dymarkowski (Department of Radiology, UZLeuven, Leuven, Belgium) for performing the CT acquisitions.

Moreover, the authors would like to thank General Electric (GE VingMed, Horten, Norway) for giving access to the 3D streaming option.

References

1. Morais, P., Vilaça, J.L., Ector, J., D'hooge, J., Tavares, J.M.R.S.: Novel solutions applied in transseptal puncture: a systematic review. J. Med. Devices **11**, 010801 (2017)
2. Hsu, J.C., Badhwar, N., Gerstenfeld, E.P., Lee, R.J., et al.: Randomized trial of conventional transseptal needle versus radiofrequency energy needle puncture for left atrial access. J. Am. Heart Assoc. **2**, e000428 (2013)
3. Jayender, J., Patel, R.V., Michaud, G.F., Hata, N.: Optimal transseptal puncture location for robot-assisted left atrial catheter ablation. Int. J. Med. Robot. Comput. Assist. Surg. **7**, 193–201 (2011)
4. Morais, P., Vilaça, J.L., Queirós, S., Marchi, A., et al.: Automated segmentation of the atrial region and fossa ovalis towards computer-aided planning of inter-atrial wall interventions. Comput. Methods Programs Biomed. **161**, 73–84 (2018)
5. Ruisi, C.P., Brysiewicz, N., Asnes, J.D., Sugeng, L., Marieb, M., Clancy, J., et al.: Use of intracardiac echocardiography during atrial fibrillation ablation. Pacing Clin. Electrophysiol. **36**, 781–788 (2013)
6. Biaggi, P., Fernandez-Golfín, C., Hahn, R., Corti, R.: Hybrid imaging during transcatheter structural heart interventions. Curr. Cardiovasc. Imaging Rep. **8**, 33 (2015)
7. Bourier, F., Reents, T., Ammar-Busch, S., Semmler, V., Telishevska, M., Kottmaier, M., et al.: Transseptal puncture guided by CT-derived 3D-augmented fluoroscopy. J. Cardiovasc. Electrophysiol. **27**, 369–372 (2016)
8. Afzal, S., Veulemans, V., Balzer, J., Rassaf, T., Hellhammer, K., Polzin, A., et al.: Safety and efficacy of transseptal puncture guided by real-time fusion of echocardiography and fluoroscopy. Neth. Heart J. **25**, 131–136 (2017)
9. Schroeder, W.J., Lorensen, B., Martin, K.: The visualization toolkit: an object-oriented approach to 3D graphics: Kitware (2004)
10. Morais, P., Tavares, J.M.R., Queirós, S., Veloso, F., D'hooge, J., Vilaça, J.L.: Development of a patient-specific atrial phantom model for planning and training of interatrial interventions. Med. Phys. **44**, 5638–5649 (2017)
11. Cleary, K., Peters, T.M.: Image-guided interventions: technology review and clinical applications. Annu. Rev. Biomed. Eng. **12**, 119–142 (2010)
12. Faletra, F.F., Biasco, L., Pedrazzini, G., Moccetti, M., et al.: Echocardiographic-fluoroscopic fusion imaging in transseptal puncture: a new technology for an old procedure. J. Am. Soc. Echocardiogr. **30**, 886–895 (2017)
13. Housden, R.J., et al.: Three-modality registration for guidance of minimally invasive cardiac interventions. In: Ourselin, S., Rueckert, D., Smith, N. (eds.) FIMH 2013. LNCS, vol. 7945, pp. 158–165. Springer, Heidelberg (2013). https://doi.org/10.1007/978-3-642-38899-6_19
14. Lang, P., Seslija, P., Chu, M.W., Bainbridge, D., Guiraudon, G.M., Jones, D.L., et al.: US–fluoroscopy registration for transcatheter aortic valve implantation. IEEE Trans. Biomed. Eng. **59**, 1444–1453 (2012)

15. Morais, P., Vilaça, J.L., Queirós, S., Bourier, F., Deisenhofer, I., Tavares, J.M.R.S., et al.: A competitive strategy for atrial and aortic tract segmentation based on deformable models. Med. Image Anal. **42**, 102–116 (2017)
16. Almeida, N., Friboulet, D., Sarvari, S.I., Bernard, O.: Left-atrial segmentation from 3-D ultrasound using b-spline explicit active surfaces with scale uncoupling. IEEE Trans. Ultrason. Ferroelectr. Frequency Control **63**, 212–221 (2016)

Holographic Visualisation and Interaction of Fused CT, PET and MRI Volumetric Medical Imaging Data Using Dedicated Remote GPGPU Ray Casting

Magali Fröhlich[1(✉)], Christophe Bolinhas[1(✉)], Adrien Depeursinge[3,4(✉)], Antoine Widmer[3(✉)], Nicolas Chevrey[2(✉)], Patric Hagmann[5(✉)], Christian Simon[6(✉)], Vivianne B. C. Kokje[6(✉)], and Stéphane Gobron[1(✉)]

[1] HE-ARC School of Engineering, University of Applied Sciences and Arts Western Switzerland (HES-SO), Neuchâtel, Switzerland
{magalistephanie.froehlich,Christophe.Bolinhas,Stephane.Gobron}@he-arc.ch
[2] HE-ARC School of Health, University of Applied Sciences and Arts Western Switzerland (HES-SO), Neuchâtel, Switzerland
Nicolas.Chevrey@he-arc.ch
[3] School of Management, University of Applied Sciences and Arts Western Switzerland (HES-SO), Sierre, Switzerland
antoine.widmer@hevs.ch
[4] Biomedical Imaging Group (BIG), Ecole polytechnique fédérale de Lausanne (EPFL), Lausanne, Switzerland
adrien.depeursinge@epfl.ch
[5] Departement of Radiology, Lausanne University Hospital (CHUV-UNIL), Rue du Bugnon 45, 1011 Lausanne, Switzerland
Patric.Hagmann@chuv.ch
[6] Departement of Otolaryngology - Head and Neck Surgery, CHUV, Lausanne, Switzerland
{Simon,Vivianne.Kokje}@chuv.ch

Abstract. Medical experts commonly use imaging including Computed Tomography (CT), Positron-Emission Tomography (PET) and Magnetic Resonance Imaging (MRI) for diagnosis or to plan a surgery. These scans give a highly detailed representation of the patient anatomy, but the usual Three-Dimensional (3D) separate visualisations on screens does not provide an convenient and performant understanding of the real anatomical complexity. This paper presents a computer architecture allowing medical staff to visualise and interact in real-time holographic fused CT, PET, MRI of patients. A dedicated workstation with a wireless connection enables real-time General-Purpose Processing on Graphics Processing Units (GPGPU) ray casting computation through the mixed reality (MR) headset. The hologram can be manipulated with hand gestures and voice commands through the following interaction features: instantaneous visualisation and manipulation of 3D scans with a frame rate of 30 fps and a delay lower than 120 ms. These performances give a seamless interactive experience for the user [10].

© Springer Nature Switzerland AG 2018
D. Stoyanov et al. (Eds.): POCUS 2018/BIVPCS 2018/CuRIOUS 2018/CPM 2018,
LNCS 11042, pp. 102–110, 2018.
https://doi.org/10.1007/978-3-030-01045-4_12

Keywords: Augmented and mixed reality · Medical application Medical visualisation · MRI scan · PET scan · CT scan GPGPU ray casting · HoloLens · Hologram

1   Introduction

Current surgical treatments rely on complex planning using traditional multiplanar rendering (MPR) of medical images including CT and MRI. The resulting imagery shows patients anatomical slices in axial, sagittal or coronal planes to plan surgery. However, details of vital internal structures are often scattered and become inconspicuous [3]. The use of 3D modeling partially solves this problem, allowing the reconstruction of patient-specific anatomy. Many studies revealed that using 3D models benefits in different surgical fields [3,8,9,11,13] improving surgical planning, shortening patient exposure time to general anaesthesia, decreasing blood loss and shortening wound exposure time. However, the visualisation and interaction of these complex 3D models on conventional environments with 2D screens remains difficult [1,3]. Indeed, user's point of view is limited by the windowing of his the screen and the manipulation via the mouse is not intuitive and a biased appreciation of distances [1,3]. This complicates clinical diagnosis and surgical planning. Today, medical data visualisation extends beyond traditional 2D desktop environments through the development Mixed Reality (MR) and Virtual Reality (VR) head-mounted displays [2,4,6,13]. These new paradigms have proven their high potential in the medical field including surgical training [6,13] and planning [3,14]. Specifically, the MR solutions have

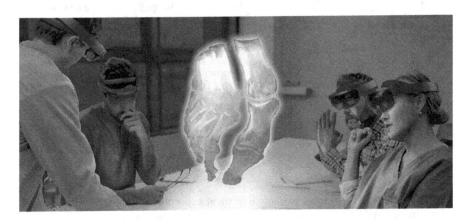

Fig. 1. This figure illustrates the potential goal: medical specialists being able to work all together on a patient dataset of fused 3D imaging modalities (MRI, PET and/or CT). The current stage of development proposes a functional solution with a single user.

already shown an interest in the problem described by displaying a personalized data visualisation [7]. Using MR, the interaction with the hologram can be at the same location as where holographic presentation is perceived [1]. This point in particular has the potential to improve surgical-planning and surgical-navigation [3,8,9,11,12]. The main goal of this paper is to describe a MR tool that displays interactive holograms of virtual organs from clinical data as illustrated in Fig. 1. With this tool, we provide a powerful means to improve surgical planning and potentially improve surgical outcome. The end-user can interact with holograms through an interface developed in this project that combines different services offered by the HoloLens.

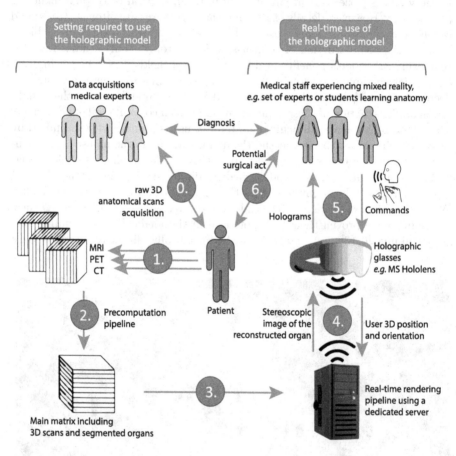

Fig. 2. Complete process from patient to medical experts using holograms to improve understanding and communication between the different actors.

2 Method and Technical Concepts

The usual pipeline used for viewing medical images in MR includes a step of pre-processed segmentation and modelisation of the medical images. The HoloLens, being an embedded system, are very far to have the processing power required to compute an advanced volumetric rendering. Therefore, a remote server with a high-end GPU to handle all the rendering processes is needed. We propose the following architecture to implement the latter is shown in Fig. 2. The process handling the volumetric rendering starts by loading the 3D scans of segmented organs in precomputation pipeline. Once the texture loaded, data are transferred to the GPU into the dedicated server and is used to render the 3D scene with all the filters and ray casting stereoscopic rendering.

Details of the rendering architecture pipeline (steps 3 to 5 of the Fig. 2) are provided in Fig. 3.

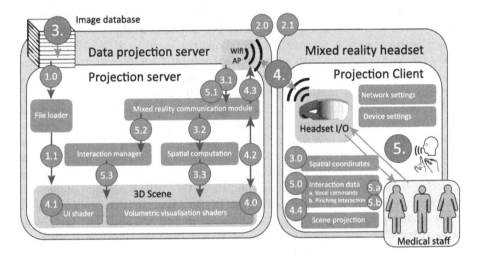

Fig. 3. Illustration of the real-time rendering pipeline.

The headset starts a remote client provided by Microsoft (MS) to receive the hologram projection so that the medical staff can visualise the data and interact in a natural manner. The headset sends back the spatial coordinates and the vocal commands to the server to update the virtual scene.

Various volumetric imaging protocols are used in clinical routine for surgical planning like CT, PET and MRI scans. Being able to mix and interact with all patient informations (volumetric anatomy as well as patient data file as floating windows) an AR setup constitutes a powerful framework for understanding and apprehending complex organ and tissue and even pathology. The proposed pre-processing pipeline could take scans as input align and encode them in a 32-bit 4096^2 matrix including segmented structures. It allowed to fuse complex structural and functional information in one single data structure stored as images in the database that can be efficiently visualised in the AR environment. The first step required to combine those scans is to resample and align them. All scans were first resampled to have 1 mm-edge length cubic volumetric pixels (voxels). The nearest neighbour interpolation was used to preserve Standardized Uptake Values SUV units in PET, whereas cubic interpolation was used for CT and MRI. The CT scan is set as a reference and both PET and MRI are mapped with a 3D translation. A second step consisted of cropping the data around the object of interest. The input of the main rendering pipeline is a 4096 × 4096 32-bits-encoded matrix. Therefore, it was first reshaped all 256^3 volumes into a 16 × 16 series of 256 adjacent axial slices to match the 4096^2 pixel format of the rendering pipeline input. Then, the PET, CT and MRI data bit depth were transformed to 8 allowing us to encode all three modalities in the first three Red, Green and Blue bytes of the 32-bits-input matrix. Since CT and PET protocols yield voxel values corresponding to absolute physical quantities, simple object segmentation can be achieved by image thresholding and morphological closing. Bone was defined as voxel values $f_{CT}(x) > 300$HU. Arteries were defined as $200 < f_{CT}(x) < 250$HU in CT images with IC. Various metabolic volumes were defined as $f_{PET}(x) > t$, where t is a metabolic threshold in SUV. All resulting binary masks were closed with a spherical structural 3 mm-diameter element to remove small and disconnected segmentation components. The binary volumes were encoded as segmentation flags in the last Alpha byte.

The real-time virtual reconstruction of body structures in voxels is done by a GPGPU massive parallel computation ray casting algorithm [5] using the preprocessed image database described. The volumetric ray casting algorithm allows to dynamically change how the data coming from the different aligned scan images are used for the final rendering. As the database described above, each rendering contains four main components: PET, CT, MRI scans and segmentation. All components are registered on an RGBα image and can be controlled in the shader parameters. The following colour modes are available: Greyscale for each layer, corresponding to the most widely used visualisation method in the medical field; Scan colour highlighting, voxel intensities within the scans and segmentation; Sliced data colouration.

Each layer can be independently controlled, filtered, colored and highlighted. Moreover, the user can change each layer aspect using ray-tracing and enhance target visualisation with segmentation highlight by changing the corresponding layer intensity. The ray casting algorithm updates the volume rendering according to the user commands: The user can quickly activate and deactivate each scan and have a perspective on the position of each body part with voice commands; The user can interact with the model in a spatial control field with the pinch command.

Geometric manipulations like rotation, scaling and translation provide a way to control the angles of the visualised hologram. This feature is essential to allow medical staff to fully use the 3D rendering and see the organic structure details. Moreover, the user can slice the 3D volume and remove data parts to focus on specific ones. Hand gestures and voice recognition algorithm voice based on MS API: MR Companion Kit.

3   Results

Results of initial testing the MR application within the Otorhinolaryngology Department of the Lausanne University Hospital (CHUV), it was concluded that the current version of the project can be applied in three different ways: (1) Greyscale image display (mostly used to plan surgery); (2) PET scan highlighted with false colours; (3) Segmentation highlighted with false colours.

The first rendering, shown in Fig. 4, is an example of a patient with a neck oropharyngeal cancer. The first image represents the mix of the three scan layers (PET, CT, and MRI) on a grey scale with a red highlight on the PET and CT. The second rendering shows the bone structure. A pink segmentation highlight is added to the 4th byte.

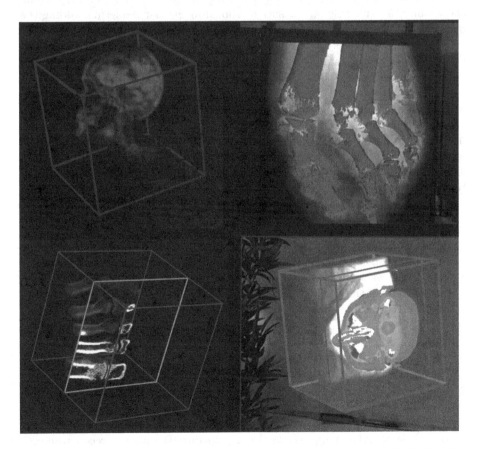

Fig. 4. Shaders implemented in this project according to use cases which display the data in different renderings. Extracted directly from the final HoloLens.

Table 1. Benchmark of different HoloLens components

Metric	Average value	Standard deviation
Frames per second	29.8 fps	±1.22 fps
Latency	119.16 ms	± 14.28 ms
HoloLens CPU Usage	46.10%	±8.07%
HoloLens GPU Engine 0	22.30%	±1.24%
HoloLens GPU Engine 1	8.69%	±0.41%
Computer CPU usage	22.67%	±5.81%
Computer GPU usage	64.50%	±9.40%
Computer RAM usage	479.52 Mo	±3.84 Mo

The third rendering shown in Fig. 4, adds a slicing functionality, which enables two kinds of renderings: one displaying a solid 2D slice and one keeping the volumetric rendering on the slice as shown in the last rendering, adding the optionality to navigate through different layers using different angles.

The current state of the application provides a proof that this concept and current material can support volumetric rendering with a dedicated server and a remote connection to the headset.

To have an estimate potential lags, a benchmark has been made with various shader models from the system as seen in Table 1. Details the average variation performance of the following functionalities: multiple-layer activation, user-finger input activation, vocal inputs, segmentation filtering, threshold filtering, scan slicing, x-ray and surface rendering as well as several colouring modes. The Table 1 certifies that immersion and hologram manipulation were very satisfying [10]. The current projects now focuses on improving the following aspects:

- Low performance when starting the remote connection;
- The remote connection resets itself if the frame reception takes too long because of packet loss;
- Frame loss during pinching inputs often leads to inaccurate manipulations;
- The above weak performance and connection reset issues will be fixed in a later version of the product. As for frame loss, improving the pipeline stability might be a suitable option.

4   Conclusion and Perspective

This paper demonstrates the high potential of fused 3D data visualising. The protocol underlines an innovative software architecture enabling real-time, practical visualisation of a massive individual patient database (i.e. 30 fps and 120 ms delay). Moreover, the manipulation of simultaneous 3D anatomic reconstructions of PET, CT and MRI allows better clinical interpretation of complex and specific 3D anatomy. The protocol can be adapted in different disciplines, not only improving surgical planning for medical professionals but also enhance surgical training and thereby increase the surgical competence for future generations.

The next step will be adding multiple users in a single 3D scene, providing a more intuitive interface, and conducting clinical indoor user tests. Feedback from users point on that one of the main remaining issue concerns the easy-to-use interface. Besides, in terms of graphical renderings, the current approach does not allow very high image resolutions but only 128^3 voxel space equivalent; currently emphasis is placed on working on a fast and more advanced version taking into account real environment with natural sphere maps.

5 Compliance with Ethical Standards

Conflict of interest – The authors declare that they have no conflict of interest.

Human and animal rights – This article does not contain any studies with human participants or animals performed by any of the authors.

References

1. Bach, B., Sicat, R., Beyer, J., Cordeil, M., Pfister, H.: The hologram in my hand: how effective is interactive exploration of 3D visualizations in immersive tangible augmented reality? IEEE TVCG **24**(1), 457–467 (2018)
2. Bernhardt, S., Nicolau, S.A., Soler, L., Doignon, C.: The status of augmented reality in laparoscopic surgery as of 2016. Med. Image Anal. **37**, 66–90 (2017)
3. Douglas, D.B., Wilke, C.A., Gibson, J.D., Boone, J.M., Wintermark, M.: Augmented reality: advances in diagnostic imaging. Multimodal Tech. Interact. **1**, 29 (2017)
4. Egger, J., et al.: HTC Vive MeVisLab integration via OpenVR for med. app. PLOS ONE **12**(3), 1–14 (2017)
5. Gobron, S., Çöltekin, A., Bonafos, H., Thalmann, D.: GPGPU computation and visualization of 3D cellular automata. Visual Comput. **27**(1), 67–81 (2011)
6. Hamacher, A., et al.: Application of virtual, augmented, and mixed reality to urology. Int. Neurourol. J. **20**(3), 172–181 (2016)
7. Karmonik, C., Boone, T.B., Khavari, R.: Workflow for visualization of neuroimaging data with an AR device. J. Digital Imaging **31**(1), 26–31 (2017)
8. Morley, C., Choudhry, O., Kelly, S., Phillips, J., Ahmed, F.. In: SIIM Scientific Session: Poster & Demostrations (2017)
9. Qian, L., et al.: Technical Note: Towards Virtual Monitors for Image Guided Interventions - Real-time Streaming to Optical See-Through Head-Mounted Displays (2017)
10. Raaen, K., Kjellmo, I.: Measuring latency in VR systems, pp. 457–462 (2015)
11. Syed, A.Z., Zakaria, A., Lozanoff, S.: Dark room to augmented reality: application of hololens technology for oral radiological diagnosis. Oral Surg. Oral Med. Oral Pathol. Oral Radiol. **124**(1), e33 (2017)
12. Tepper, O.M., et al.: Mixed reality with HoloLens. Plast. Reconstr. Surg. **140**(5), 1066–1070 (2017)

13. Vaughan, N., Dubey, V.N., Wainwright, T.W., Middleton, R.G.: A review of virtual reality based training simulators for orthopaedic surgery. Med. Eng. Phys. **38**(2), 59–71 (2016)
14. Wang, J., et al.: Real-time computer-generated integral imaging and 3D image calibration for augmented reality surgical navigation. Comput. Med. Imaging Graph. **40**, 147–159 (2015)

Mr. Silva and Patient Zero: A Medical Social Network and Data Visualization Information System

Patrícia C. T. Gonçalves[1,2(✉)], Ana S. Moura[3],
M. Natália D. S. Cordeiro[3], and Pedro Campos[1,4]

[1] LIAAD - Laboratório de Inteligência Artificial e Apoio à Decisão,
INESC TEC - Instituto de Engenharia de Sistemas e Computadores,
Tecnologia e Ciência, 4200-465 Porto, Portugal
pctg@inesctec.pt

[2] Departamento de Engenharia e Gestão industrial, Faculdade de Engenharia,
Universidade do Porto, 4200-465 Porto, Portugal

[3] LAQV-REQUIMTE, Departamento de Química e Bioquímica,
Faculdade de Ciências, Universidade do Porto, 4169-007 Porto, Portugal

[4] Departamento de Matemática e Sistemas de Informação,
Faculdade de Economia, Universidade do Porto, 4200-465 Porto, Portugal

Abstract. Detection of Patient Zero is an increasing concern in a world where fast international transports makes pandemia a Public Health issue and a social fear, in cases such as Ebola or H5N1. The development of a medical social network and data visualization information system, which would work as an interface between the patient medical data and geographical and/or social connections, could be an interesting solution, as it would allow to quickly evaluate not only individuals at risk but also the prospective geographical areas for imminent contagion. In this work we propose an ideal model, and contrast it with the *status quo* of present medical social networks, within the context of medical data visualization. From recent publications, it is clear that our model converges with the identified aspects of prospective medical networks, though data protection is a key concern and implementation would have to seriously consider it.

Keywords: Medical social networks · Data visualization · Epidemiology

1 Introduction

Global epidemic outbreaks are increasing in frequency and social concern, with recent proposals focusing on global and transversal possible solutions to act with speed and feasibility in the development of vaccines and therapeutics [1]. However, another issue is essential in approaching global or local epidemiological outbreaks, which is the sure and fast identification of Patient Zero. This identification matters because: (a) knowing the medical history of the first individual to become infected with the pathogen and, thus, becoming the first human infectious vehicle, can help determine the initial conditions of the outbreak; (b) it can also indicate the original non-human source of the

© Springer Nature Switzerland AG 2018
D. Stoyanov et al. (Eds.): POCUS 2018/BIVPCS 2018/CuRIOUS 2018/CPM 2018,
LNCS 11042, pp. 111–117, 2018.
https://doi.org/10.1007/978-3-030-01045-4_13

epidemiological context; and (c) the knowledge of the primordial exposure allows for the epidemiologists to acquire precision on the 'who', 'where', 'how' and 'when' of the outbreak.

Nevertheless, we cannot resist to quote David Heymann, of the London School of Hygiene & Tropical Medicine, when he says that the search for Patient Zero is paramount as long as they still disseminate the disease as a living focus, which, for most of the occasions, does not happen [2]. And it is regarding this latter, the localization of Patient Zero still alive, that the use of medical social networks may be invaluable.

What we call a medical social network is a medical-based application of the principles of social networks. Barabási, one of the pioneers of medical social networks, wrote that networks can be found on every particulars and features of human health [3]. However complex the relationship between the network individuals, the organizing principles are attainable through graph theory and visualization, namely as nodes and edges [4]. In a medical context, the nodes may represent biological factors, which can be as diverse as diseases or phenotypes, and the edges represent any chosen relationship, from physical interaction to shared trait. In the field of Epidemiology, for instance, the nodes can be infected individuals, and the edges the physical interactions between them. Albeit this simplification, other aspects can be added (e.g., distinguish between female and male individuals while maintaining the infected information – *vide* Fig. 1). This fusion between social networks and medicine may allow for the detection of patterns of symptomatology, within a community, of public health interest.

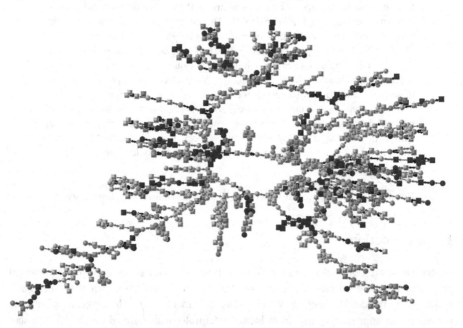

Fig. 1. Example of a medical social network. Each node represents a person - circles denote women, and squares men. Node colour denotes happiness: blue indicating the least happy, and yellow the happiest (green are intermediate). Black edges represent siblings' relationship, and red edges denote friendship or spouses. [Adapted from [5], courtesy of the authors]. (Color figure online)

With the purpose of reviewing the *status quo* of medical networks and data visualization within this context, the present work is divided into the following sections. In Sect. 2, we discuss an ideal medical network model and how feasible it would be dealing with the above mentioned issues. In Sect. 3, selected medical/health network models are discussed in transversal analysis and contrasted with the ideal model. Finally, our conclusions are summarized while also pointing out several prospective paths regarding the development of future medical social networks.

2 Ideal Information System

Let us consider the following hypothetical scenario. I am a doctor and am about to meet Mr. Silva, my patient. Prior to his entering, I access all the data he has given me permission to. In this ideal medical Information System (IS), along with Mr. Silva's standard clinical data (blood tests results, X-ray images, doctor's appointments records, etc.), I also have access to the following social network data: (a) Mr. Silva's kinship network of, at least, two degree relatives (i.e., first degree relatives such as parents, siblings, or offspring, and second degree relatives, such as uncles, aunts, grandparents or full cousins), and their medical data relevant for Mr. Silva's current health condition; (b) through a user friendly interface, I can change the data shown on the network, choosing the information that I see fit; (c) red alerts on medical networks, national and/or local, regarding Mr. Silva's personal connections, that is, connections within a workplace or neighbourhood context. The importance of these outputs lies on cross-referencing Mr. Silva's family medical history with his social interactions.

This ideal IS's purpose is not only to aid physicians during their consultations and serve as a decision support for their diagnoses, but also to act as a disease prevention and public health tool. For that, a work team of skilled IT analysts and managers, data scientists, and health professionals from different areas, will be constantly working with this IS, analyzing all the continuous outputs it provides, namely: (a) different medical social networks illustrating various types of links, such as the family connections between people with a certain medical condition on a certain geographical location, or the working connections between people of a certain age interval that present certain symptoms; (b) alerts for potential health threats already ongoing or as a measure of prevention of those threats. Using this medical IS, this work team should provide frequent reports on the state of the population health regarding all kinds of diseases, and, of course, immediately inform the reporting hierarchies of any and all alerts.

To achieve these outputs, the input of this medical Information System consists of: (a) all administrative data, such as patients full name and address, workplace address, and direct contact number; (b) identification of all the patient's direct relatives, up to the second degree (at least); (c) the physicians' consultations records.

Still in the scope of prevention and treatment of diseases, access to some of these data, and even the use of some of the IS functionalities, may be requested by researchers under official research projects.

Patients' anonymity is of major importance, and even during Mr. Silva's consultation his doctor will only know the type of relationship Mr. Silva has with the people in his social network(s), and their clinical data. Further, the protected data could allow for network pattern and community detection without exposing the identity of the patients, which would be invaluable not only for long-term Public Health measures but also Emergency Management. Regarding public interest, the identity of the connections would only be known in cases of severe gravity and, cumulatively, with external authorization. This would take into account the legal and ethical right of the patient to privacy.

3   Medical Social Networks: The General State of Affairs

Having described the ideal medical IS, we now proceed to discuss the present and general state of affairs of medical social networks.

To begin with, there is not, to our knowledge, a formal medical IS that incorporates social network analysis, but there are several published models which can point out the present capacity, possible implementation and likely reception of a formal medical IS based on them. As such, a selection of those models, chosen due to the specific details that can enhance a cross-reference and discussion with our proposed ideal model, are presented by chronological order and their transversal comparison made by table data displaying and discussion.

Table 1 presents the specifics for identifying the selected models, indicating per row the year of publication, the authors, the subject and the type of sample. The time-span covered by the selected models belongs to the period 2012–2017, and the cultural context presents a wide variety from the USA, to Honduras and India. The subjects approach both physical and emotional aspects of medical social networks, i.e., the models can address, as portrayed in Fig. 1, psychological/sociological aspects of the individuals as components of their overall health situation. Table 2 summarizes the main conclusions and type of data visualization per study.

Table 1. Medical networks' models from recent years.

Study	Year	Subject	Sample
[6]	2012	Aspirin use and cardiovascular events in social networks	2,724 members of the Framingham Heart Study, Massachusets, USA
[7]	2014	Association between social network communities and health behaviour	16,403 individuals in 75 villages in rural Karnataka, India
[8]	2015	Social network targeting to maximise population behaviour change	Individuals aged 15 or above recruited from villages of the Department of Lempira, Honduras
[9]	2017	Association of Facebook use with compromised well-being	5,208 subjects in the Gallup Panel Social Network Study survey, USA

Strully *et al.* depart from a simple interrogation: if the adoption of aspirin of a social element after a cardiovascular event would affect the adoption of aspirin intake as a preventive measure by his/hers social circle [6]. Using a longitudinal logistic regression

Table 2. Medical networks data visualization

Study	Data visualization	Conclusions
[6]	Table with results with columns per statistical functions	- Predisposition for daily intake of aspirin if a social connection presented such routine - Absence of individual discrimination per social network can bias the conclusions
[7]	Table with results of multilevel logistic regression analysis AND network depiction of a village	- Suggestion of organic social network communities more strongly associated with normatively driven behaviour than with direct or geographical social contacts - Norm-based interventions could be more effective if they target network communities within villages
[8]	Network depiction of a block of villages	- Friend targeting increased adoption of the nutritional intervention - Suggestion that network targeting can efficiently be used to ensure the success of certain types of public health interventions
[9]	Table with results from multivariate regression analysis AND box/whisker plots	- The associative process between Facebook use and compromised well-being is dynamic - Suggestion that, overall, Facebook use may not promote well-being

model, and three waves from data extracted from the Framingham Heart Study, they defined as dependent variable the daily intake of aspirin by the individual at the time of the wave. The interest lay if the daily basis intake of aspirin was common in the three waves and, if not, if there was a cardiovascular incident of a social connection that could explain that change. The model considered several aspects of the individuals (e.g., gender or type of social connection) and the results were displayed on tables, with statistical functions, such as average percentage, confidence intervals or adjusted odds ratio. The display of data did not allow a visualization of each individual specific 'decision environment', *i.e.*, conclusions are drawn for the population but the individual aspects become elusive. The authors commented that, although they detected the sharing of the doctor as a common feature to change in aspirin intake habits, the data did not allow knowing whether the doctors actively influenced it. In fact, the authors stated that one of the limitations of their research was the lack of randomness, which may have introduced some homophily-driven selection bias, based on unobserved characteristics that may influence the use of aspirin over time, such as drug addiction.

The study conducted by Shakya *et al.* applied an algorithmic social network method to several Indian village communities to explore not only possible connection between latrine ownership and community-level and village-level latrine ownership, but also the degree to which network cohesion affected individual latrine ownership [7]. The authors used a social network depiction to contrast with the statistical results and concluded more strongly regarding the effect of connections in influencing the change in health habits (in this case, ownership of latrine), even stating that one could consider such network understanding a new field of research, which would debunk large data sets analysis into health policies intelligibility and its subsequent efficiency on daily practices.

In 2015, Kim *et al.* evaluated with network-based approaches which methods maximise population-level behaviour change, considering interventions on several health areas (e.g. nutrition), and considered the results evidenced the network-based approach had the advantage of being independent from previous network mapping [8]. Further, they considered that network-based models could sustain the development of health policies intended to change the individual routines, albeit more research should be conducted to discriminate which of the targeting methods presented better adequacy to different classes of interventions.

Our final selected publication deals with the eventual effects of social media network use and well-being. Shakya and Christakis assessed the potential effects of both online and real-world social networks, cross referencing the respondent's direct Facebook data and real-world social networks self-reported data for a longitudinal association in four domains of well-being [9]. They point out that the longitudinal data was size limited due to a small number of permissions to access Facebook data and that the models, though consistent in the direction and magnitude of some associations, did not identify the mechanisms between Facebook use and reduced well-being.

Cross-referencing these models with our ideal medical Information System, it is clear that: (1) data visualization may be the difference between general and non-elusive conclusions; (2) medical social network models are becoming transversal and accepted to understand, identify and be part of the solution of several medical issues; and (3) data protection needs to be carefully implemented for the success of the ideal medical IS.

4 Conclusions and Future Perspectives

Regarding prevention, it is paramount to have a medical tool allowing us to screen the social network of the patient, as it can identify certain health issues per geographical region and per social interaction. Though location of Patient Zero is important in a national crisis, non-epidemiological diseases, such as depression, can present contagion as well and are the silent epidemics. A medical social network as we suggest can locate these silent Patient Zeros and promote overall successful Public Health policies and individual well-being and support.

Acknowledgments. Patrícia C. T. Gonçalves and Pedro Campos would like to thank the European Regional Development Fund (ERDF) through the COMPETE 2020 Programme, project POCI-01-0145-FEDER-006961, and the National Funds through the Fundação para a Ciência e a Tecnologia (FCT) as part of project UID/EEA/50014/2013. Ana S. Moura and M. Natalia D.S. Cordeiro acknowledge the support by Fundação para a Ciência e a Tecnologia

(FCT/MEC) through national funds and co-financed by FEDER, under the partnership agreement PT2020 (Projects UID/MULTI/50006 and POCI-01-0145-FEDER-007265).

References

1. Carroll, D., et al.: The Global Virome Project. Science **359**, 872–874 (2018)
2. Mohammadi, D.: Finding patient zero. Pharm. J. 294(**7845**) (2015). https://doi.org/10.1211/PJ.2015.20067543
3. Barabási, A.-L.: Network medicine — from obesity to the "Diseasome". N. Engl. J. Med. **357**, 404–407 (2007)
4. Newman, M.E.J.: Networks: An Introduction. Oxford University Press, Oxford (2010)
5. Christakis, N.A., Fowler, J.H.: Social network visualization in epidemiology. Nor. Epidemiol. (Nor. J. Epidemiol.) **19**, 5–16 (2009)
6. Strully, K.W., Fowler, J.H., Murabito, J.M., Benjamin, E.J., Levy, D., Christakis, N.A.: Aspirin use and cardiovascular events in social networks. Soc. Sci. Med. **74**, 1125–1129 (2012)
7. Shakya, H.B., Christakis, N.A., Fowler, J.H.: Association between social network communities and health behavior: an observational sociocentric network study of latrine ownership in rural India. Am. J. Public Health **104**, 930–937 (2014)
8. Kim, D.A., et al.: Social network targeting to maximise population behaviour change: a cluster randomised controlled trial. Lancet **386**, 145–153 (2015)
9. Shakya, H.B., Christakis, N.A.: Association of Facebook use with compromised well-being: a longitudinal study. Am. J. Epidemiol. **185**, 203–211 (2017)

Fully Convolutional Network-Based Eyeball Segmentation from Sparse Annotation for Eye Surgery Simulation Model

Takaaki Sugino[1]([✉]), Holger R. Roth[1], Masahiro Oda[1], and Kensaku Mori[1,2,3]

[1] Graduate School of Informatics, Nagoya University, Nagoya, Japan
tsugino@mori.m.is.nagoya-u.ac.jp
[2] Information Technology Center, Nagoya University, Nagoya, Japan
[3] Research Center for Medical Bigdata, National Institute of Informatics, Tokyo, Japan

Abstract. This paper presents a fully convolutional network-based segmentation method to create an eyeball model data for patient-specific ophthalmologic surgery simulation. In order to create an elaborate eyeball model for each patient, we need to accurately segment eye structures with different sizes and complex shapes from high-resolution images. Therefore, we aim to construct a fully convolutional network to enable accurate segmentation of anatomical structures in an eyeball from training on sparsely-annotated images, which can provide a user with all annotated slices if he or she annotates a few slices in each image volume data. In this study, we utilize a fully convolutional network with full-resolution residual units that effectively learns multi-scale image features for segmentation of eye macro- and microstructures by acting as a bridge between the two processing streams (residual and pooling streams). In addition, a weighted loss function and data augmentation are utilized for network training to accurately perform the semantic segmentation from only sparsely-annotated axial images. From the results of segmentation experiments using micro-CT images of pig eyeballs, we found that the proposed network provided better segmentation performance than conventional networks and achieved mean Dice similarity coefficient scores of 91.5% for segmentation of eye structures even from a small amount of training data.

Keywords: Segmentation · Fully convolutional networks Eyeball modeling · Sparse annotation · Micro CT

1 Introduction

Semantic segmentation of medical images is an essential technique for creating anatomical model data that are available for surgical planning, training,

© Springer Nature Switzerland AG 2018
D. Stoyanov et al. (Eds.): POCUS 2018/BIVPCS 2018/CuRIOUS 2018/CPM 2018,
LNCS 11042, pp. 118–126, 2018.
https://doi.org/10.1007/978-3-030-01045-4_14

and simulation. In the field of ophthalmology, elaborate artificial eyeball models [1,2] have been developed for training and simulation of eye surgeries, and it is desired to create realistic eyeball model data for patient-specific surgical simulation through the segmentation of detailed eye structures. Thus, we focus on segmenting not only the entire eyeball structure but also microstructures (e.g., Zinn's zonule) in the eyeball, which conventional modalities such as computed tomography (CT) have difficulty capturing, by using higher-resolution modalities such as micro CT.

To efficiently create patient-specific eyeball model data from high-resolution images, we need to take into account the following three points: (a) full- or semi-automation of segmentation for reducing the burden of manual annotation, (b) accurate extraction of eye structures with different sizes and complex shapes, and (c) image processing at full resolution without downsampling. Therefore, we utilize a fully convolutional network (FCN) [3], which is one of the most powerful tools for end-to-end semantic segmentation, to construct a segmentation method to fulfill the key points.

For accurate segmentation of objects with different sizes and complex shapes in the images, it is important to construct a network architecture that can obtain image features for localization and recognition of the objects. In general, deep convolutional neural networks can obtain coarse image features for recognition on deep layers and fine image features for localization on shallow layers. Many studies [3–6] have proposed a network architecture to obtain multi-scale image features for semantic segmentation by residual units (RUs) or skip connections, which combine different feature maps output from different layers. U-net proposed by Ronneberger et al. [6] achieved good performance for semantic segmentation of biomedical images by effectively using long-range skip connections. Moreover, their research group showed that 3D U-net [7], which was developed as the extended version of U-net, could provide accurate volumetric image segmentation based on training from sparsely-annotated images on three orthogonal planes. However, such 3D FCNs have difficulty handling images at full resolution and obtaining full-resolution image features essential for strong localization performance because of the limitation of GPU memory.

Therefore, we aim to construct a 2D network architecture that provides improved localization and recognition for semantic segmentation of high-resolution medical images by using advanced RUs instead of conventional skip connections found in FCN-8s [3] or U-net [6]. Moreover, we also aim to propose a training strategy in which the network can learn from sparsely-annotated images and provide accurate label propagation to the remaining images in volumetric image data, because it is not easy to collect a large amount of high-resolution image volumes for network training from different cases. The concept of our proposed method is shown in Fig. 1. The originality of this study lies in introducing a FCN with the advanced RUs and its training strategy to achieve accurate segmentation of eye structures in an end-to-end fashion even from sparsely-annotated volumetric images.

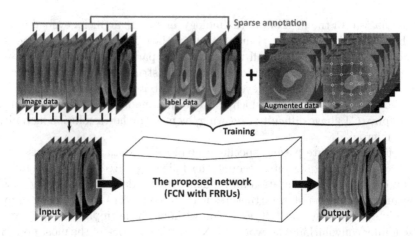

Fig. 1. Concept of the proposed method for segmentation of eye structures from sparse annotation

2   Methods

2.1   Network Architecture

In this study, we focus on full-resolution residual units (FRRUs) [8], which was designed to facilitate the combination of multi-scale image features while keeping similar training characteristics as ResNet [9]. We utilize the network architecture that consists of four pooling steps followed by four upsampling steps like U-net [6] as a base and construct a residual-based FCN incorporating FRRUs into the basal network architecture to enhance the localization and recognition performances for segmentation of eye structures. Figure 2 shows the architectures of U-net and the proposed network. The box in the figure represents a feature map output by each convolution layer or FRRU and the number of channels is denoted under the box. U-net fuses the same-size feature maps between pooling stages and upsampling stages with skip connections, while the proposed network jointly computes image features on two processing streams by using FRRUs. One stream (i.e., residual stream) conveys full-resolution fine image features for localization, which are obtained by adding successive residuals, and the other stream (i.e., pooling stream) conveys coarse image features for recognition, which are computed through convolution and pooling steps.

The detail of a FRRU structure is indicated in Fig. 3. Each classical RU [9] has one input and one output, while each FRRU computes two outputs from two inputs. Let x_n and y_n be the residual and the pooling inputs to n-th FRRU, respectively. Then, the outputs are computed as follows:

$$x_{n+1} = x_n + \mathcal{G}(x_n, y_n; W_n) \tag{1}$$

$$y_{n+1} = \mathcal{H}(x_n, y_n; W_n) \tag{2}$$

where W_n denote the parameters of the residual function $\mathcal{G}$ and the pooling function $\mathcal{H}$. As shown in Fig. 3, the FRRU concatenates the pooling input with the residual input operated by a pooling layer, and subsequently obtains the concatenated features (i.e., the output of the function $\mathcal{H}$) through two 3×3 convolution layers. The output of $\mathcal{H}$ is passed to the next layer as the pooling stream. Moreover, the output of $\mathcal{H}$ are also resized by the function $\mathcal{G}$ and reused as features added to the residual stream. This design of the FRRU makes it possible to combine and compute the two stream simultaneously and successively.

Therefore, the proposed network, which are composed of a sequence of FRRUs, gains the ability to precisely localize and recognize objects in images by combining the following two processing streams: the residual stream that carries fine image features at full resolution and the pooling stream that carries image features obtained through a sequence of convolution, pooling, and deconvolution operations.

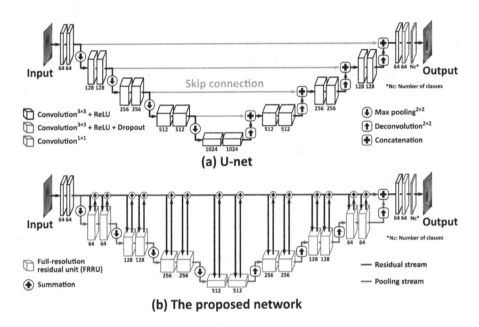

Fig. 2. Network architectures: (a) U-net [6] and (b) the proposed network

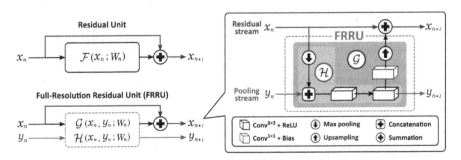

Fig. 3. Design of full-resolution residual unit (FRRU) [8]

2.2 Training Strategy

We assume that the proposed network is applied to eye structures segmentation based on sparse annotation. Thus, we need to construct a framework to enable the network to effectively learn image features even from less annotated slices for training.

In the case of our application, it is expected that the training and testing subsets of images have no significant differences of geometric and visual characteristics (e.g., location, scale, or contrast) between objects for segmentation because they are derived from the same image volume. Therefore, we here adopt rotation and elastic deformation for data augmentation to efficiently train small geometric variations of eye structures in the images based on less annotated slices for training, although there are many techniques for increasing the amount of training data. Each slice in the training subset is augmented twentyfold by rotating $-25°$ to $25°$ at 5 degree intervals and repeating the elastic deformation ten times based on random shifts of 5×5 grid points and B-spline interpolation.

Additionally, for more effective network training, we use categorical cross-entropy loss function weighted by the inverse of class frequency to reduce the negative effects of class imbalance (i.e., difference of sizes between different eye structures in the images).

3 Experiments and Results

3.1 Experimental Setup

We validated the segmentation performance of the proposed method on a dataset of eyeball images, which were scanned using a micro-CT scanner (inspeXio SMX-90CT Plus, Shimadzu Co., Japan). The dataset consists of micro-CT volumes of five pig eyeballs, and the size of each volume is $1024 \times 1024 \times 548$ (sagittal $\times$ coronal $\times$ axial) voxels, with a voxel size of 50 µm. Figure 4 shows an example of micro-CT images and label images used for the validation. As a preprocessing step, the original micro-CT images were filtered by using a wavelet-FFT filter [10] and a median filter to remove the ring artifacts and random noises, and subsequently the filtered images were normalized based on the mean and standard deviation on the training subset of images for each micro-CT volume. We defined six labels, including Background, Wall and membrane, Lens, Vitreum, Ciliary body and Zinn's zonule, and Anterior chamber. The preprocessed images and the corresponding manually annotated images were used for network training and testing.

In this study, for fundamental comparative evaluation, we compared our network with the following two representative networks: FCN-8s [3] and U-net [6]. To evaluate the segmentation performances associated with network architectures, all the networks were trained and tested on the same datasets under the same conditions (i.e., the same learning rate, optimizer, and loss function were assigned to the networks). On the assumption of the semantic segmentation from

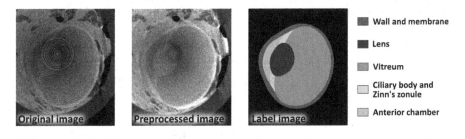

Fig. 4. Example of micro-CT images and label images

sparse annotation, 2.5% (i.e., every 40 slices) of all the slices and the remaining slices on the axial plane in each volume were used as training and testing subsets, respectively. The slices of each training subset were augmented by the two data augmentation techniques (i.e., rotation and elastic deformation). Each of the networks was trained from scratch on the augmented training subset of slices for 100 epochs and tested on the testing subset. The segmentation performances were quantitatively and qualitatively evaluated by comparing Dice similarity coefficient (DSC) scores and visualization results between the networks. The networks used for experiments were implemented using Keras[1] with the Tensorflow backend[2], and all the experiments were performed on a NVIDIA Quadro P6000 graphic card with 24 GB memory.

3.2   Experimental Results

Table 1 indicates the comparison results of DSC scores of the three networks, including FCN-8s, U-net, and the proposed network. The proposed network could segment eye structures with a mean Dice score of 91.5% and achieve the best segmentation performance of the three networks. In addition, the results showed that the proposed network could segment almost all the labels with higher mean score and lower standard deviation than the other networks. Even on the label of "Ciliary body & Zinn's zonule" that is hard to segment because of the high variability of shapes, the proposed network provided mean DSC score of more than 85%.

Figure 5 visualizes a part of the segmentation results obtained by the three networks. FCN-8s generalized the segmentation results with jagged edges near the label boundaries, and U-net produced segmentation results including some errors despite the smooth label boundaries. Compared to these conventional networks, we could find that the proposed network generalized more accurate segmentation results with smoother edges for all labels than the other networks.

---

[1] https://keras.io/.

[2] https://www.tensorflow.org/.

Table 1. Quantitative comparison of segmentation results of pig eyeballs ($n = 5$)

Label	DSC score (%)		
	(a) FCN-8s[3]	(b) U-net[6]	(c) Our network
Background	99.7 ± 0.2	99.7 ± 0.1	**99.8 ± 0.1**
Wall and membrane	83.2 ± 6.1	86.9 ± 3.4	**89.4 ± 1.4**
Vitreum	**97.8 ± 0.4**	96.9 ± 1.4	97.8 ± 0.8
Lens	94.4 ± 1.9	94.3 ± 1.4	**95.5 ± 1.1**
Ciliary body & Zinn's zonule	79.7 ± 6.4	82.9 ± 3.1	**85.6 ± 2.8**
Anterior chamber	87.5 ± 4.9	85.3 ± 4.7	**89.1 ± 1.9**
Mean (except Background)	88.5	89.3	**91.5**
Std (except Background)	7.6	6.2	**5.1**
Min (except Background)	79.7	82.9	**85.6**
Max (except Background)	**97.8**	96.9	**97.8**

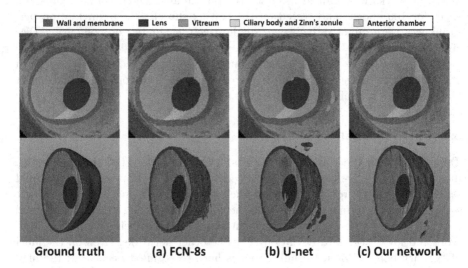

Ground truth   (a) FCN-8s   (b) U-net   (c) Our network

Fig. 5. Qualitative comparison of segmentation results

4   Discussion

As indicated in Table 1, the proposed network achieved high mean DSC scores
with low standard deviation for segmenting eye structures from sparse annotation, although only 2.5% of all the slices (i.e., 14 of 548 slices) were used for
network training. The proposed network could consistently achieve higher accuracy for segmentation of eye structures with different sizes and shapes, compared
to FCN-8s and U-net. This is probably because the proposed network succeeded
in learning more robust image features against the change of sizes and shapes in

the images. In other words, these results imply a FRRU contributes to obtaining finer features for strong localization.

In addition, Fig. 5 showed that the proposed network could generalize segmentation results with more accurate and smoother class boundaries compared to FCN-8s and U-net, although it produced some false positives. This can be considered to be due to the fact that the loss of fine image features occurred in the training process, especially in the pooling operations. Although both of them had skip connections for obtaining multi-scale features, it is probably difficult to convey image features for precise localization by only the conventional skip connections. Therefore, the network architecture incorporating FRRUs can be very effective to learn multi-scale image features, which conventional architectures have difficulty capturing.

However, even the network with FRRUs failed to provide accurate segmentation results on some slices. Thus, in future work, we will aim to further improve the segmentation accuracy of our network by combining other strategies for obtaining multi-scale image features (e.g., dilated convolutions [11]), and then we will apply our network to segmentation of finer eye structures from higher-resolution images such as X-ray refraction-contrast CT images [12] to create more elaborate eyeball model.

5   Conclusion

In this study, we proposed a FCN architecture and its training scheme for segmenting eye structures from high-resolution images based on sparse annotation. The network architecture consists of a sequence of FRRUs, which enable to effectively combine multi-scale image features for localization and recognition. Experimental results on micro-CT volumes of five pig eyeballs showed that the proposed network outperformed conventional networks and achieved mean segmentation accuracy of more than 90% by training with the weighted loss function on the augmented data, even from very few annotated slices. The proposed segmentation method may have the potential to help create an eyeball model for patient-specific eye surgery simulation.

Acknowledgments. Parts of this work were supported by the ImPACT Program of Council for Science, Technology and Innovation (Cabinet Office, Government of Japan), the JSPS KAKENHI (Grant Numbers 26108006, 17K20099, and 17H00867), and the JSPS Bilateral International Collaboration Grants.

References

1. Joag, M.G., et al.: The bioniko ophthalmic surgery model: an innovative approach for teaching capsulorhexis. Investig. Ophthalmol. Vis. Sci. **55**(13), 1295–1295 (2014)
2. Someya, Y., et al.: Training system using bionic-eye for internal limiting membrane peeling. In: 2016 International Symposium on Micro-NanoMechatronics and Human Science (MHS), pp. 1–3. IEEE (2016)
3. Long, J., Shelhamer, E., Darrell, T.: Fully convolutional networks for semantic segmentation. In: IEEE Conference on Computer Vision and Pattern Recognition, pp. 3431–3440 (2015)
4. Badrinarayanan, V., Kendall, A., Cipolla, R.: Segnet: a deep convolutional encoder-decoder architecture for image segmentation. IEEE Trans. Pattern Anal. Mach. Intell. **39**(12), 2481–2495 (2017)
5. Lin, G., Milan, A., Shen, C., Reid, I.: Refinenet: multi-path refinement networks for high-resolution semantic segmentation. In: IEEE Conference on Computer Vision and Pattern Recognition, pp. 1925–1934 (2017)
6. Ronneberger, O., Fischer, P., Brox, T.: U-Net: convolutional networks for biomedical image segmentation. In: Navab, N., Hornegger, J., Wells, W.M., Frangi, A.F. (eds.) MICCAI 2015. LNCS, vol. 9351, pp. 234–241. Springer, Cham (2015). https://doi.org/10.1007/978-3-319-24574-4_28
7. Çiçek, Ö., Abdulkadir, A., Lienkamp, S.S., Brox, T., Ronneberger, O.: 3D U-Net: learning dense volumetric segmentation from sparse annotation. In: Ourselin, S., Joskowicz, L., Sabuncu, M.R., Unal, G., Wells, W. (eds.) MICCAI 2016. LNCS, vol. 9901, pp. 424–432. Springer, Cham (2016). https://doi.org/10.1007/978-3-319-46723-8_49
8. Pohlen, T., Hermans, A., Mathias, M., Leibe, B.: Full-resolution residual networks for semantic segmentation in street scenes. In: IEEE Conference on Computer Vision and Pattern Recognition, pp. 4151–4160 (2017)
9. He, K., Zhang, X., Ren, S., Sun, J.: Deep residual learning for image recognition. In: IEEE Conference on Computer Vision and Pattern Recognition, pp. 770–778 (2016)
10. Münch, B., Trtik, P., Marone, F., Stampanoni, M.: Stripe and ring artifact removal with combined wavelet-Fourier filtering. Opt. Express **17**(10), 8567–8591 (2009)
11. Yu, F., Koltun, V.: Multi-scale context aggregation by dilated convolutions. In: International Conference on Learning Representations (ICLR) (2016)
12. Sunaguchi, N., Yuasa, T., Huo, Q., Ichihara, S., Ando, M.: X-ray refraction-contrast computed tomography images using dark-field imaging optics. Appl. Phys. Lett. **97**(15), 153701 (2010)

International Workshop on Correction of Brainshift with Intra-Operative Ultrasound, CuRIOUS 2018

Resolve Intraoperative Brain Shift
as Imitation Game

Xia Zhong[1(✉)], Siming Bayer[1], Nishant Ravikumar[1], Norbert Strobel[4],
Annette Birkhold[2], Markus Kowarschik[2], Rebecca Fahrig[2],
and Andreas Maier[1,3]

[1] Pattern Recognition Lab, Friedrich-Alexander University
Erlangen-Nürnberg, Erlangen, Germany
xia.zhong@fau.de
[2] Siemens Healthcare GmbH, Forchheim, Germany
[3] Erlangen Graduate School in Advanced Optical Technologies (SAOT),
Erlangen, Germany
[4] Fakultät für Elektrotechnik, Hochschule für angewandte Wissenschaften
Würzburg-Schweinfurt, Würzburg and Schweinfurt, Germany

Abstract. Soft tissue deformation induced by craniotomy and tissue
manipulation (*brain shift*) limits the use of preoperative image overlay
in an image-guided neurosurgery, and therefore reduces the accuracy of
the surgery as a consequence. An inexpensive modality to compensate
for the brain shift in real-time is Ultrasound (US). The core subject of
research in this context is the non-rigid registration of preoperative MR
and intraoperative US images. In this work, we propose a learning based
approach to address this challenge. Resolving intraoperative brain shift
is considered as an imitation game, where the optimal action (displacement) for each landmark on MR is trained with a multi-task network.
The result shows a mean target error of 1.21 ± 0.55 mm.

1 Introduction

In a neurosurgical procedure, the exposed brain tissue undergoes a time dependent elastic deformation caused by various factors, such as cerebrospinal fluid
leakage, gravity and tissue manipulation. Conventional image-guided navigation
systems do not take any elastic brain deformation (*brain shift*) into account.
Consequently, the neuroanatomical overlays produced prior to the surgery does
not correspond to the actual anatomy of the brain without an intraoperative
image update. Hence, real-time intraoperative brain shift compensation has a
great impact on the accuracy of image-guide neurosurgery.

An inexpensive modality to update the preoperative MRI image is Ultrasound (US). Its intraoperative repeatability offers another further benefit with
respect to real-time visualization of intra-procedural anatomical information [1].
Both feature- and intensity-based deformable, multi-modal (MR-US) registration approaches are proposed to perform brain shift compensation.

D. Stoyanov et al. (Eds.): POCUS 2018/BIVPCS 2018/CuRIOUS 2018/CPM 2018,
LNCS 11042, pp. 129–137, 2018.
https://doi.org/10.1007/978-3-030-01045-4_15

In general, brain shift compensation approaches are based on feature-driven deformable registration methods to update the preoperative images by establishing correspondence of selected homologous landmarks. Performance of Chamfer Distance Map [2], Iterative Closest Point (ICP) [3] and Coherent Point Drift [4] are evaluated in phantom [2,4] and clinical studies [3]. Inherently, the accuracy of feature-based methods is limited by the quality of the landmark segmentation and feature mapping algorithm.

Intensity-based algorithms overcome these intrinsic problems in the feature-based methods. Similarity metrics such as sum of squared differences [5] and normalized mutual information [6] were first proposed to register preoperative MR and iUS non-rigidly. However, intensity-based US-MR non-rigid registration poses a significant challenge due to the low signal-to-noise ratio (SNR) of the ultrasound images and different image characteristics and resolution of US and MR images. To tackle this challenge, Arbel et al., [7] first generates a pseudo US image based on the preoperative MR data and performs US-US non-rigid registration by optimizing the normalized Cross Correlation metric. Recently, local correlation ratio was proposed in a PaTch-based cOrrelation Ratio (RaPTOR) framework [8], where preoperative MR was registered to postresection US for the first time.

Recent advances in reinforcement learning (RL) and imitation learning (or behavior cloning) encourages the reformulation of the MR-US non-rigid registration problem. Krebs et al. [9] trained an artificial agent to estimate the Q-value for a set of pre-calculated actions. Since the Q-value of an action effects the current and future registration accuracy, a sequence of deformation fields for optimal registration can be estimated by maximizing the Q-value. In general, reinforcement learning presupposes a finite set of reasonable actions and learns the optimal policy to predict a combinatorial action sequence of the finite set. However, in a real world problem such as intraoperative brain shift correction, the number of feasible actions are infinite. Consequently, reinforcement learning is hardly to be adapted to resolve brain shift. In contrast, imitation learning is proposed to learn the actions itself. To this end, an agent is trained to mimics the action taken by the demonstrator in associated environment. Therefore, there is no restriction on the number of the actions. It has been used to solve tasks in robotic [10] and autonomous driving systems [11]. Our previous work reformulated the organ segmentation problem as imitation learning and showed good result [12].

Inspired by Turing's original formulation of imitation game, we reformulate the brain shift correction problem based on the theory of imitation learning in this work. A multi-task neural network is trained to predict the movement of the landmarks directly by mimicking the ground-truth action exhibits by the demonstrator.

2   Imitation Game

We consider the registration of a preoperative MRI volume to the intraoperative ultrasound (iUS) for brain-shift correction as an imitation game. The game is constructed by first defining the environment. The environment $\mathbb{E}$ for the brain-shift correction using registration is defined as the underlying iUS volume and MRI volume. The key points $\boldsymbol{P}^{\mathbb{E}} = [\boldsymbol{p}_1^{\mathbb{E}}, \boldsymbol{p}_2^{\mathbb{E}}, \cdots \boldsymbol{p}_N^{\mathbb{E}}]^T$ in the MRI volume are shifted non-rigidly in three-space to target points $\boldsymbol{Q}^{\mathbb{E}} = [\boldsymbol{q}_1^{\mathbb{E}}, \boldsymbol{q}_2^{\mathbb{E}}, \cdots, \boldsymbol{q}_N^{\mathbb{E}}]^T$ in the iUS volume. Subsequently, we define the demonstrator as a system able to estimate the ideal action, in the form of a piece-wise linear transformation $\boldsymbol{a}_i^{\mathbb{E},t}$, for the ith key point $\boldsymbol{p}_i^{\mathbb{E},t}$, in the tth observation $\boldsymbol{O}^{\mathbb{E},t}$, to the corresponding target point $\boldsymbol{q}_i^{\mathbb{E},t}$. The goal of the game is defined as the act of finding an agent $\mathcal{M}(\cdot)$, to mimic the demonstrator and predict the transformations of the key points given an observation. This was formulated as a least square problem (Eq. 1).

$$\arg\min_{\mathcal{M}} = \sum_{\mathbb{E}} \sum_{t} \|\mathcal{M}(\boldsymbol{O}^{\mathbb{E},t}) - \boldsymbol{A}^{\mathbb{E},t}\|_2^2 \tag{1}$$

Here, $\boldsymbol{A}^{\mathbb{E},t} = [\boldsymbol{a}_1^{\mathbb{E},t}, \boldsymbol{a}_2^{\mathbb{E},t}, \cdots, \boldsymbol{a}_N^{\mathbb{E},t}]^T$ denotes the action of all N key points. In the context of brain shift correction, we use annotated landmarks in the MRI as key points $\boldsymbol{p}_i^t$ and landmarks in iUS as target points $\boldsymbol{q}_i^t$. A neural network is employed as our agent $\mathcal{M}$.

2.1   Observation Encoding

We encode the observation of the point cloud in the environment as a feature vector. For each point $\boldsymbol{p}_i^{\mathbb{E},t}$ in the point cloud, we extract a cubic sub-volume centered at this point in three-space. The cubic sub-volume has an isotropic dimension of C^3 and voxel size of S^3 in mm and its orientation is identical to the world coordinate system. The value of each voxel in the sub-volume is extracted by sampling the underlying iUS volume in the corresponding position, and interpolating using trilinear interpolation. We denote the sub-volume encoding as a matrix $\boldsymbol{V}^{\mathbb{E},t} = [\boldsymbol{v}_1^{\mathbb{E},t}, \boldsymbol{v}_2^{\mathbb{E},t}, \cdots \boldsymbol{v}_N^{\mathbb{E},t}]^T$, where each sub-volume is flattened into a vector $\boldsymbol{v}_i^{\mathbb{E},t} \in \mathbb{R}^{C^3}$. Apart from the sub-volume, we also encode the point cloud information into the observation. We normalized the point cloud to a unit sphere and used the normalized coordinates $\tilde{\boldsymbol{P}}^{\mathbb{E},t} = [\tilde{\boldsymbol{p}}_1^{\mathbb{E},t}, \tilde{\boldsymbol{p}}_2^{\mathbb{E},t}, \cdots, \tilde{\boldsymbol{p}}_N^{\mathbb{E},t}]^3$ as a part in the encoding. The observation $\boldsymbol{O}^{\mathbb{E},t}$ is a concatenation of $\boldsymbol{V}^{\mathbb{E},t}$ and $\tilde{\boldsymbol{P}}^{\mathbb{E},t}$.

2.2   Demonstrator

The demonstrator predicts the action $\boldsymbol{A}^{\mathbb{E},t} \in \mathbb{R}^{3 \times N}$ of the key points. We define the action for brain shift as the displacement vector for the key points to move to their respective targets. As both the target points and the key points are known, one intuitive way to calculate the action for each key point is to compute the displacement field directly as $\boldsymbol{a}_i^{\mathbb{E},t} = \boldsymbol{q}_i^{\mathbb{E},t} - \boldsymbol{p}_i^{\mathbb{E},t}$. As we can see, this demonstrator estimates the displacement independent of the observation. This can make the learning difficult. Therefore, we also calculate the translation vector $\boldsymbol{t}_i^{\mathbb{E},t} = \bar{\boldsymbol{q}}_i^{\mathbb{E},t} - \bar{\boldsymbol{p}}_i^{\mathbb{E},t} \in \mathbb{R}^{3 \times 1}$ as the auxiliary output of the demonstrator. Hence, the objective function is,

$$\arg\min_{\mathcal{M}} = \sum_{\mathbb{E}} \sum_{t} \|\mathcal{M}(\boldsymbol{O}^t) - \boldsymbol{A}^t\|_2^2 + \lambda\|\mathcal{M}'(\boldsymbol{O}^t) - \boldsymbol{t}^t\|_2^2 \qquad (2)$$

where, $\mathcal{M}'$ denotes the agent estimating the auxiliary output and λ is the weighting of the auxiliary output. In the implementation, a multi-task neural network is implemented as both $\mathcal{M}$ and $\mathcal{M}'$.

2.3   Data Augmentation

To facilitate the learning process, we augment the training dataset to increase the number of samples and the overall variability. In the context of brain shift correction, data augmentation can be applied both to the environment $\mathbb{E}$ and to the key points $\boldsymbol{P}^{\mathbb{E},t}$. In order to augment the environment $\mathbb{E}$, the elastic deformation proposed by Simard et al. [13] is applied to the MRI and iUS volumes. Varieties of brain shift deformations are simulated by warping the T1, flair MRI volumes and the iUS volume, together with their associated landmarks, independently, using two different deformation fields.

In each of the augmented environments, we also augmented the key points' (MRI landmarks) coordinates in two different ways. For each key point, we added a random translation vector with a maximal magnitude of 1 mm in each direction. This synthetic non-rigid deformation was included to mimic interrater differences that may be included, during landmark annotation [14]. An additional translation vector was also used to shift all key points with a maximal magnitude of 6 mm in each direction. This was done to simulate the residual rigid registration error introduced during the initial registration using fiducial markers. Of particular importance, is how these augmentation steps were applied to the data. We assumed the translation between the key points and target points in the training data to be a random registration error. Consequently, we initially aligned the key points to the center of gravity of the target points. The center of gravity is defined as mean of all associated points. The non-rigid and translation augmentation steps were applied subsequently, to the key points.

2.4   Imitation Network

As observation encoding and the demonstrator are both based on a point cloud, the imitation network also works with a point cloud. Inspired by PointNet [15], which process the point cloud data without a neighborhood assumption efficiently, we proposed a network architecture that utilizes both the known neighborhood in the sub-volume $\boldsymbol{V}^{\mathbb{E},t}$, and the unknown permutation of associated key points $\tilde{\boldsymbol{P}}^{\mathbb{E},t}$. The network is depicted in Fig. 1. The network uses the sub-volume and key points as two inputs and processes them independently. During observation encoding, each row vector denotes a sub-volume $\boldsymbol{v}_i^{\mathbb{E},t} \in \mathbb{R}^{C^3}$ of the associated key point $\boldsymbol{p}_i^{\mathbb{E},t}$. Therefore, we use three consecutive $C \times 1$ convolutions with a stride size of $C \times 1$, to approximate a 3D separable convolution and extract the texture feature vectors. We also employ 3×1 convolution kernels to extract features from key points. These low-level features are concatenated for

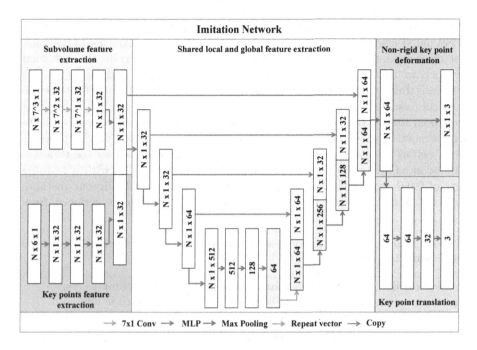

Fig. 1. Illustration imitation network architecture.

further processing. The main part of the network largely employs the PointNet architecture, where we use a multilayer perceptron (MLP) to extract local features, and max pooling to extract global features. The local and global features are concatenated to propagate the gradient and facilitate the training process. The multi-task learning formulation of the network also helps improves overall robustness. We used batch normalization for each layer and ReLU as activation function. One property of the network is that if a copy of a key point and a associated sub-volume is added as additional input, the output of the network for these key points remains unchanged. This is especially useful in the context of brain-shift correction, where the number of key points usually varies before and after resection. Therefore, we use the maximum number of landmarks in the training data as input key point number of our network. For a training data smaller than this number, we arbitrarily copy one of the key points. Finally, after predicting the deformation of the key points, the deformation field between them is interpolated using B-splines.

3   Evaluation

We trained and tested our method using the Correction of Brainshift with Intra-Operative Ultrasound (CuRIOUS) MICCAI challenge 2018 data. This challenge use the clinical dataset described in [14]. In the current phase of the challenge, 23 datasets are used as training data, in which 22 comprise the required MRI and ultrasound landmark annotations before dura opening. The registration method is evaluated using target registration error (mTRE) in mm. We used leave-one-out cross-validation to train and evaluate our method. To train the imitation network, we used 19 datasets for training, two for validation and one as the test set. Each training and validation dataset was augmented by 32 folds for the environment cascaded with 32 folds key points augmentation. In total 19.4k datasets were used for the training, 2k were used for validation. We chose a sub-volume with isometric dimensions $C = 7$ and voxel size of $2 \times 2 \times 2 \, \text{mm}^3$. 16 points were used as input key points and a batch size of 128 was used for the training. The adapted Adam optimizer proposed by Sashank et al. [16] with a learning rate of 0.001 was used. The results are shown in Table 1. Using our method, the overall mean target registration errors (mTREs) can be reduced from

Table 1. Evaluation of the mean distance between landmarks in MRI and ultrasound before and after correction.

Patient ID	Landmarks number	Mean distance (range) initial in mm	Mean distance (range) corrected in mm
1	15	1.82 (0.56–3.84)	0.88 (0.25–1.39)
2	15	5.68 (3.43–8.99)	1.01 (0.42–2.32)
3	15	9.58 (8.57–10.34)	1.10 (0.30–4.57)
4	15	2.99 (1.61–4.55)	0.89 (0.25–1.58)
5	15	12.02 (10.08–14.18)	1.78 (0.66–5.05)
6	15	3.27 (2.27–4.26)	0.72 (0.27–1.26)
7	15	1.82 (0.22–3.63)	0.86 (1.72–0.28)
8	15	2.63 (1.00–4.15)	1.45 (0.73–2.40)
12	16	19.68 (18.53–21.30)	2.27 (1.17–4.31)
13	15	4.57 (2.73–7.52)	0.96 (0.31–1.44)
14	15	3.03 (1.99–4.43)	0.87 (0.31–1.92)
15	15	3.32 (1.15–5.90)	0.69 (0.23–1.17)
16	15	3.39 (1.68–4.47)	0.83 (0.34–1.96)
17	16	6.39 (4.46–7.83)	0.96 (0.31–1.61)
18	16	3.56 (1.44–5.47)	0.89 (0.33–1.33)
19	16	3.28 (1.30–5.42)	1.26 (0.41–1.74)
21	16	4.55 (3.44–6.17)	0.85 (0.26–1.33)
23	15	7.01 (5.26–8.26)	1.08 (0.28–3.40)
24	16	1.10 (0.45–2.04)	1.61 (0.52–2.84)
25	15	10.06 (7.10–15.12)	1.76 (0.62–1.76)
26	16	2.83 (1.60–4.40)	0.93 (0.47–1.44)
27	16	5.76 (4.84–7.14)	2.88 (0.79–5.45)
Mean ± STD		5.37 ± 4.27	1.21 ± 0.55

$5.37 \pm 4.27\,\text{mm}$ to $1.21 \pm 0.55\,\text{mm}$. In a similar setting, but applied to different datasets, the state-of-the-art registration method RaPTOR has an overall mTRE of $2.9 \pm 0.8\,\text{mm}$ [8].

The proposed imitation network has 0.22 M trainable parameters, requires 6.7 M floating point operations (FLOPS), and converges within 7 epochs. To calculate the computational complexity in the application phase, we consider the network having a complexity of $\mathcal{O}(1)$ due to pretraining. The observation encoding step has a complexity of $\mathcal{O}(N \times C^3)$, where N denotes the number of key points and C denotes the number of sub-volume dimension. Therefore, the complexity of the proposed algorithm is $\mathcal{O}(N \times C^3)$, independent of the resolution of underlying MRI or iUS volume. In the current implementation, the average runtime of the algorithm is $1.77\,\text{s}$, of which 88% time is used for observation encoding using CPU.

4 Discussion

To our best knowledge, an imitation learning based approach is proposed for the first time in the context of brain shift correction. The presented method achieves encouraging results within $2\,\text{mm}$ with real-time capability ($<2\,\text{s}$). In 21 out of 22 datasets, the mTREs are reduced significantly. As the mTRE in 22th dataset is initially small, the inter-rater difference of $0.5\,\text{mm}$ is still remarkable [14]. Hence, these results indicates the applicability of the proposed method in the clinical environment. However, following aspects should be concerned for the further development. One important aspect is the number and variation of the training data used in the proposed imitation learning algorithm. Although the number of the training datasets are increased effectively by applying data augmentation methods (described in Sect. 2.3), variation of the training data such as location of the tumor and orientation of the head cannot be augmented without further considerations. A common tool to simulate the different image orientation is rotational augmentation. However, it alters the effect of gravity implicitly, therefore results in unrealistic training data. Thus, rotational augmentation is inappropriate for the data augmentation in context of brain shift compensation. The other aspect is the comprehensive validation of the proposed method. The generalizability and robustness should be evaluated with a larger amount of data acquired with different intraoperative image modalities. In this challenge, we use landmarks as key points and predict the deformation of the landmarks directly. In future applications, we could also adapt our approach to control points of a free-form deformation or contour points of a certain structure (e.g. vessel). The associated target points could be either manually annotated or automatically estimated with point matching algorithms.

5 Conclusion

In this study, we proposed a novel approach for intra-operative brain shift correcting, during tumor resection surgery, using imitation learning. The presented method uses observation encoding to describe the local texture and point-cloud information and the trained imitation network is used to estimate the movement of landmarks defined in pre-operative MR volumes, directly to their counterparts in iUS volumes, based on this encoding. Our network reduced the mean landmark distance between the pre- and intra-operative image pairs substantially, from $5.37 \pm 4.27\,\text{mm}$ to $1.21 \pm 0.55\,\text{mm}$, in real-time, which is particularly compelling for its future use in a surgical setting. Additionally, the proposed approach is flexible, as it is not modality- or anatomy-specific, and thus could be employed in a variety of image-guided surgical interventions.

References

1. Bayer, S., Maier, A., Ostermeier, M., Fahrig, R.: Intraoperative imaging modalities and compensation for brain shift in tumor resection surgery. Int. J. Biomed. Imaging **2017** (2017)
2. Reinertsen, I., Descoteaux, M., Drouin, S., Siddiqi, K., Collins, D.L.: Vessel driven correction of brain shift. In: Barillot, C., Haynor, D.R., Hellier, P. (eds.) MICCAI 2004. LNCS, vol. 3217, pp. 208–216. Springer, Heidelberg (2004). https://doi.org/10.1007/978-3-540-30136-3_27
3. Reinertsen, I., Lindseth, F., Unsgaard, G., Collins, D.L.: Clinical validation of vessel-based registration for correction of brain-shift. Med. Image Anal. **11**(6), 673–684 (2007)
4. Farnia, P., Ahmadian, A., Khoshnevisan, A., Jaberzadeh, A., Serej, N.D., Kazerooni, A.F.: An efficient point based registration of intra-operative ultrasound images with MR images for computation of brain shift; a phantom study. In: IEEE EMBC 2011, pp. 8074–8077, August 2011
5. Pennec, X., Cachier, P., Ayache, N.: Tracking brain deformations in time-sequences of 3D US images. Pattern Recognit. Lett. **24**(4–5), 801–813 (2003)
6. Letteboer, M.M.J., Willems, P.W.A., Viergever, M.A., Niessen, W.J.: Non-rigid registration of 3D ultrasound images of brain tumours acquired during neurosurgery. In: Ellis, R.E., Peters, T.M. (eds.) MICCAI 2003. LNCS, vol. 2879, pp. 408–415. Springer, Heidelberg (2003). https://doi.org/10.1007/978-3-540-39903-2_50
7. Arbel, T., Morandi, X., Comeau, R.M., Collins, D.L.: Automatic non-linear MRI-ultrasound registration for the correction of intra-operative brain deformations. Comput. Aided Surg. **9**, 123–136 (2004)
8. Rivaz, H., Chen, S.S., Collins, D.L.: Automatic deformable MR-ultrasound registration for image-guided neurosurgery. IEEE Trans. Med. Imaging **34**(2), 366–380 (2015)
9. Krebs, J., et al.: Robust non-rigid registration through agent-based action learning. In: Descoteaux, M., Maier-Hein, L., Franz, A., Jannin, P., Collins, D.L., Duchesne, S. (eds.) MICCAI 2017. LNCS, vol. 10433, pp. 344–352. Springer, Cham (2017). https://doi.org/10.1007/978-3-319-66182-7_40
10. Argall, B.D., Chernova, S., Veloso, M., Browning, B.: A survey of robot learning from demonstration. Robot. Auton. Syst. **57**(5), 469–483 (2009)
11. Bojarski, M., et al.: End to end learning for self-driving cars. arXiv preprint arXiv:1604.07316 (2016)
12. Zhong, X., et al.: Action learning for 3D point cloud based organ segmentation. arXiv preprint arXiv:1806.05724 (2018)

13. Simard, P.Y., Steinkraus, D., Platt, J.C., et al.: Best practices for convolutional neural networks applied to visual document analysis. In: ICDAR, vol. 3, pp. 958–962 (2003)
14. Xiao, Y., Fortin, M., Unsgård, G., Rivaz, H., Reinertsen, I.: REtroSpective Evaluation of Cerebral Tumors (RESECT): a clinical database of pre-operative MRI and intra-operative ultrasound in low-grade glioma surgeries. Med. Phys. **44**, 3875–3882 (2017)
15. Qi, C.R., Su, H., Mo, K., Guibas, L.J.: Pointnet: deep learning on point sets for 3D classification and segmentation. Proc. IEEE Comput. Soc. Conf. Comput. Vis. Pattern Recognit. **1**(2), 4 (2017)
16. Reddi, S.J., Kale, S., Kumar, S.: On the convergence of adam and beyond. In: International Conference on Learning Representations (2018)

Non-linear Approach for MRI to intra-operative US Registration Using Structural Skeleton

Jisu Hong[1] and Hyunjin Park[2,3(✉)]

[1] Department of Electronic, Electrical and Computer Engineering,
Sungkyunkwan University, Suwon, Korea
bal25ne@skku.edu
[2] School of Electronic Electrical Engineering,
Sungkyunkwan University, Suwon, Korea
hyunjinp@skku.edu
[3] Center for Neuroscience Imaging Research (CNIR),
Institute for Basic Science, Suwon, Korea

Abstract. Gliomas are primary brain tumors of central nervous system. Appropriate resection of gliomas in the early tumor stage is known to increase survival rate. However, the accurate resection of tumor is a challenging problem because the soft tissue shift may occur during the operation. To provide proper guidance to neurosurgery, it is necessary to align magnetic resonance imaging (MRI) and intra-operative ultrasound (iUS). In previous studies, many algorithms tried to find fiducial points that can lead to the appropriate registration. But these methods required manual specifications from experts to ensure the reliability of the fiducials. In this study, we proposed a data-driven approach for MRI-iUS non-linear registration using structural skeletons. The visualization of our results indicated that our approach might provide better registration performance.

Keywords: MRI · intra-operative US · Registration · Skeleton

1 Introduction

Gliomas are primary brain tumors of central nervous system (CNS) [1]. The gliomas arise from the glia which supports the CNS and can permeate to the neighboring areas. They can be categorized in grade from I to IV based on their histological characteristics defined by the World Health Organization (WHO) [2]. The grade I and II gliomas are classified as low-grade gliomas (LGG) and grade III and IV gliomas are classified as high-grade gliomas (HGG). The LGG grow comparatively slowly but due to their infiltrative attribute and threatening behavior, the mean 10-year survival is 30% [1]. It is generally accepted that the resection of the LGG may increase the survival rate [3].

Intra-operative ultrasound (iUS) was first proposed as a potential tool for guiding resection of intracranial tumors in 1980 [4]. The iUS is still generally used because it enables the surgeons to track the brain tissues and surgical tools in a fast, inexpensive, and real-time way. In addition, the gliomas can often be detected in iUS images even

© Springer Nature Switzerland AG 2018
D. Stoyanov et al. (Eds.): POCUS 2018/BIVPCS 2018/CuRIOUS 2018/CPM 2018,
LNCS 11042, pp. 138–145, 2018.
https://doi.org/10.1007/978-3-030-01045-4_16

when they are not detectable under the microscope. This can promote accurate resection and helps to obtain better surgical results. However, it is difficult to design effective surgical plans without the high-quality image-guidance. One of the principal reason is that the surgical target and the other tissues can be shifted by intra-operative factors such as tissue removal, change of intracranial pressure and drug administration. However, these shifts may not be easily observed in the surgeon's field of view.

To estimate and rectify for spatial errors resulting from intra-operative brain shifts, registration of pre-operative magnetic resonance imaging (MRI) to iUS image has been suggested [5–7]. This approach helps updating the surgical plans under the continuous brain tissue shift in contrast to comparing directly between pre- and intra-operative images. Many algorithms for registration have been proposed in the past years. However, it is technically demanding because of its intrinsic limits such as the differences between modalities and image qualities. Because of these problems, most MRI to iUS registration methods were conducted by using manually selected fiducial points.

In this paper, we proposed an automatic non-linear MRI-iUS registration algorithm using structural skeletons. First, we conducted several pre-processing steps on the MRI and iUS. Then we calculated the structural skeletons of both modalities. Finally, we calculated the displacement fields using the pairs of skeleton for the MRI-iUS registration.

2 Materials and Methods

2.1 Dataset

As this proposal is submitted to the CURIOUS 2018 challenge, we used the Retrospective Evaluation of Cerebral Tumors (RESECT) dataset [8]. The dataset includes pre-operative 3T MRI images including Gadolinium-enhanced T1w and T2 FLAIR scans, iUS images as a 3D volume covering the entire tumor region after craniotomy but before dura opening and the expert-labeled homologous anatomical landmarks, defined on all image modalities. All reconstructed images were acquired from the same subject and were spatially aligned under the same world coordinate space.

The MR protocol included T1w Gadolinium-enhanced sequence (TE = 2.96 ms, TR = 2000 ms, 192 slices, slice thickness = 1 mm, acquisition matrix = 256 × 256, in-plane resolution = 1.0 × 1.0 mm^2) and FLAIR sequence (TE = 388 ms, TR = 5000 ms, 192 slices, slice thickness = 1 mm, acquisition matrix = 256 × 256, in-plane resolution = 1.0 × 1.0 mm^2), acquired on a 3T MRI scanner with a 20-channel head coil. For subject 2, 14, 15 (Case 2, 14, 15), the pre-operative MRI included T1w sequence (TE = 2.3 ms, TR = 2500 ms, 176 slices, slice thickness = 1 mm, acquisition matrix = 512 × 496, in-plane resolution = 1.0 × 1.0 mm^2) and FLAIR sequence (TE = 333 ms, TR = 6000 ms, 176 slices, slice thickness = 1 mm, acquisition matrix = 256 × 224, in-plane resolution = 1.0 × 1.0 mm^2) acquired on a 1.5T MRI scanner with a 12-channel head coil.

The iUS images were acquired using the Sonowand Invite neuronavigation system. In most cases, the 12FLA-L linear probe with a frequency range of 6 to 12 MHz and a footprint of 48×13 mm^2 was used. For smaller tumors, the 12FLA flat linear array probe with a frequency range of 6 to 12 MHz and a footprint of 32×11 mm^2 was used. The resolution of reconstructed 3D volume varied from $0.14 \times 0.14 \times 0.14$ mm^3 to $0.24 \times 0.24 \times 0.24$ mm^3 depending on the probe types and imaging depth.

2.2   MRI Pre-processing

First, we corrected non-uniformity to remove field bias from the MRI image. After the bias removal, we obtained the masks of grey matter (GM), white matter (WM) and cerebrospinal fluid (CSF) from the T1w image. After that, we cropped the T1w image and its masks to match with the location and size of iUS image. Then we resampled the cropped image and masks into $0.2 \times 0.2 \times 0.2$ mm^3 voxel resolution. Because the intensity distribution of iUS image was well matched with the GM and CSF mask from the MRI image, we used the inversed WM mask instead of using the summation of GM and CSF mask. The small hole of the inversed mask was removed using flood-fill algorithm with connectivity parameter 4 per each z-slice. The output mask was used to calculate the structural skeleton of MRI image.

2.3   iUS Pre-processing

We resampled the iUS image using the cropped and resampled T1w image as reference. As the voxel resolution of reference image was $0.2 \times 0.2 \times 0.2$ mm^3, the iUS image resampled to the same resolution. The order of axis in iUS image was matched with the reference image. Then, the resampled iUS image was blurred with 0.5 mm full width at half maximum (FWHM) Gaussian kernel and filtered with $3 \times 3 \times 3$ median kernel under voxel coordinate space. A binary mask image was obtained by applying threshold to the filtered image and was dilated by the ball shaped structure elements with voxel radius 15. The dilated mask was used for calculating the skeleton. We used a semi-automatic intensity-based segmentation algorithm to compute the binary masks for both MRI and iUS. The masks were structurally enhanced using preprocessing steps such as full with half maximum smoothing and morphological operations, which was performed with typical hyperparameters.

2.4   Structural Skeleton

After the refinement of the binary masks, the Euclidean skeletons were calculated for both masks [9, 10]. For details, we inverted the masks and computed the Euclidean distance map. The ridges of the distance map were computed by watershed algorithm. The final skeletons of each masks were obtained by thresholding the gradient of the ridges.

2.5 Registration Using Deformation Fields

We applied the Demon's algorithm for non-linear registration [11]. This algorithm performed over the entire space of displacement field. At first, a spatial transformation field was initialized. Then, we iterated the following steps until the error converged:

(1) Given field s, compute a correspondence update field u by minimizing the error E which can be defined as following Eq. (1).

$$E(u) = ||F - M \cdot (s + u)||^2 + \left(\frac{\sigma_i}{\sigma_x}\right)||u||^2 \qquad (1)$$

(2) Let c as $s + u$.
(3) Use diffusion-like regularization by conducting the Gaussian smoothing to the accumulated transformation field c
(4) Substitute s with the filtered c.

As mentioned above, the variable s accounts for the given spatial transformation field and u for the corresponding update field. The variable F accounts for the fixed iUS image, M for the moving MRI image, σ_i for the noise on the image intensity and σ_x for a spatial uncertainty on the correspondences.

2.6 Mean Target Registration Error

We measured the Euclidean distances between the MRI landmarks after the registration and the corresponding iUS landmarks to calculate the target registration errors (TREs). All landmarks were averaged per each case.

3 Results

3.1 Crop and Resampling

Figure 1 shows the results images after cropping and resampling. Figure 1(a) and (b) represent the T1w image and the iUS image respectively. Both images were well aligned to each other so that they could be used for the following processes.

3.2 Estimated Skeleton

Cropped and resampled MRI and iUS images were used to calculate their structural skeletons. Figure 2 shows the skeletons obtained from the MRI and iUS images. Figure 2(a) shows the MRI image and its skeleton, and Fig. 2(b) shows the iUS image and its skeleton.

3.3 Skeleton Registration Using Displacement Fields

Figure 3 shows the results of the registration using the Demon's deformation algorithm. Figure 3(a) shows the original skeleton of the MRI image. Figure 3(b) and

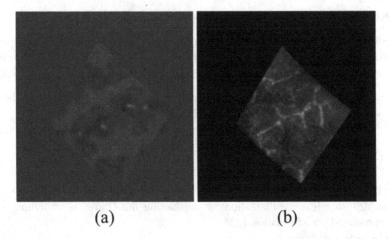

(a)   (b)

Fig. 1. The MRI image and iUS image obtained after crop and resampling of case 1. (a) is the MRI image and (b) is the iUS image.

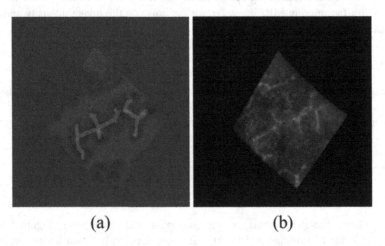

(a)   (b)

Fig. 2. The MRI image and iUS image of case 1 with their structural skeleton. (a) The structural skeleton of the MRI was indicated with green line and (b) the structural skeleton of the iUS was indicated with red line. (Color figure online)

(c) represents the deformation fields along x-axis, top-to-bottom axis in this image, and y-axis, left-to-right axis in this image respectively. The deformation field along z-axis was also calculated but it was not shown in this figure for better visualization. Figure 3 (d) is the skeleton of the MRI image after the registration to iUS image. We compared these results with the original iUS image and its skeleton (Fig. 4). The skeleton of the iUS image was shown as the structural line with red color on both Fig. 4(a) and (b). The structural line with green color on Fig. 4(a) represents the skeleton of MRI image before the registration and the same line on Fig. 4(b) represents the skeleton after the registration.

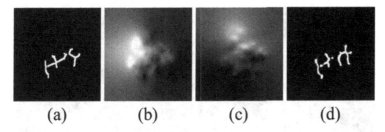

Fig. 3. The results of the registration using the Demon's deformation algorithm. (a) is the original skeleton of MRI. (b) and (c) shows the displacement field estimated after the registration on the x-axis and the y-axis respectively. (d) is the skeleton of MRI after the MRI-iUS registration.

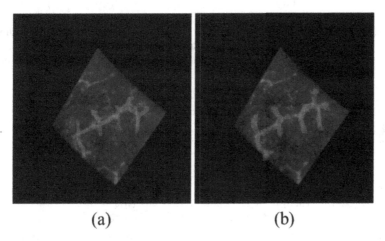

Fig. 4. The demonstration of the registration using skeletons overlapped on the same iUS image of case 1. (a) shows the skeleton of original MRI with red line and the skeleton of iUS image with green line. (b) shows the skeleton of registered MRI with red line and the skeleton of iUS image with green line. (Color figure online)

3.4   Image Registration Using Estimated Fields

As we calculated the deformation fields at each location on every axis, we could obtain the final registered MRI image (Fig. 5). Figure 5(a) shows the original MRI image overlapped with the iUS image. The MRI image was visualized with the green color and the iUS image was visualized with red color. Figure 5(b) shows the registered MRI image overlapped with the iUS image.

3.5   Landmark Evaluation

The Euclidean distances between two corresponding landmarks were measured. Then, the mTREs of all cases were measured to evaluate the results (Table 1).

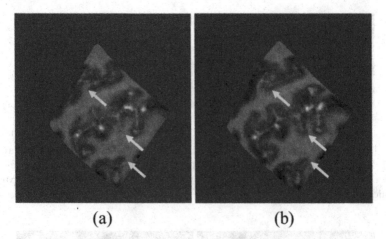

(a)   (b)

Fig. 5. The demonstration of the registration. (a) The MRI image before the registration was shown as green and the original iUS image was shown as red. (b) The MRI image after the registration was shown as green and the original iUS was shown as red. (Color figure online)

Table 1. The mean target registration error for the all 22 cases.

Case	Mean target before-registration error (mm)	Mean target after-registration error (mm)
1	1.8196	3.1779
2	5.6755	5.8900
3	9.5772	9.6980
4	2.9859	3.9038
5	12.0191	11.7075
6	3.2696	2.4846
7	1.8190	3.3739
8	2.6344	3.3612
12	19.6793	17.9112
13	4.5716	3.9380
14	3.0322	3.3116
15	3.2115	5.0273
16	3.3909	3.3728
17	6.3939	7.7679
18	3.5604	3.5396
19	3.2805	4.0459
21	4.5463	3.5659
23	7.1108	5.9944
24	1.1011	1.7430
25	10.0601	11.6948
26	2.8339	2.1951
27	5.7560	5.5233
Mean ± SD	5.38 ± 4.27	5.60 ± 3.94

References

1. Shields, L.: Management of low-grade gliomas: a review of patient-perceived quality of life and neurocognitive outcome. World Neurosurg. **87**(1–2), 299–309 (2014)
2. Louis, D.N.: The 2016 World Health Organization classification of tumors of the Central Nervous System: a summary. Acta Neuropathol. **131**(6), 803–820 (2016)
3. Asgeir, S.: Comparison of a strategy favoring early surgical resection vs a strategy favoring watchful waiting in low-grade gliomas. JAMA **308**(18), 1881–1888 (2012)
4. Voorhies, R.M.: Preliminary experience with intraoperative ultrasonographic localization of brain tumors. Radiol. Nucl. Med. **10**, 8–9 (1980)
5. Hill, D.L.: Medical image registration. Phys. Med. Biol. **46**(3), R1–R45 (2001)
6. Sotiras, A.: Deformable medical image registration: a survey. IEEE Trans. Med. Imaging **32**, 1153–1190 (2013)
7. Schnabel, J.A.: Advances and challenges in deformable image registration: from image fusion to complex motion modelling. Med. Image Anal. **33**, 145–148 (2016)
8. Xiao, Y.: REtroSpective Evaluation of Cerebral Tumors (RESECT): a clinical database of pre-operative MRI and intra-operative ultrasound in low-grade glioma surgeries. Med. Phys. **44**(7), 3875–3882 (2017)
9. Couprie, M.: Topological maps and robust hierarchical Euclidean skeletons in cubical complexes. Comput. Vis. Image Underst. **117**(4), 355–369 (2013)
10. Telea, A.: An augmented fast marching method for computing skeletons and centerlines. In: Proceedings of the symposium on Data Visualization, pp. 251–259. Eurographics, Aire-la-Ville (2002)
11. Vercauteren, T., Pennec, X., Perchant, A., Ayache, N.: Non-parametric diffeomorphic image registration with the demons algorithm. In: Ayache, N., Ourselin, S., Maeder, A. (eds.) MICCAI 2007. LNCS, vol. 4792, pp. 319–326. Springer, Heidelberg (2007). https://doi.org/10.1007/978-3-540-75759-7_39

Brain-Shift Correction with Image-Based Registration and Landmark Accuracy Evaluation

Wolfgang Wein[✉]

ImFusion GmbH, Munich, Germany
wein@imfusion.de

Abstract. We describe an algorithm and its implementation details for automatic image-based registration of intra-operative ultrasound to MRI for brain-shift correction during neurosurgery. It is evaluated on a public database of 22 surgeries for retrospective evaluation, with a particular focus on choosing the appropriate transformation model and designing the most meaningful evaluation strategy. The method succeeds in a fully automatic fashion in all cases, with an average landmark registration error for the rigid model of 1.75 mm.

1 Introduction

For brain tumor resection, navigated surgery is an established approach, allowing for pre-operative MRI images and planned structures to be available during surgery, registered to various intra-operative tools by means of an external tracking system. However, the accuracy of such systems is often affected by changing soft tissue throughout the course of surgery. Intra-operative 3D freehand ultrasound, tracked with the same localizer than the other surgical tools, allows for updated information about the resection site during all stages of surgery. Unfortunately, only surgeons who are also expert users of medical ultrasound embrace this approach currently. For it to be more widely used and applicable, more automatic handling of the intra-operative ultrasound is crucial. In particular, automatic image-based registration of the 3D ultrasound data to pre-operative MRI is a first important prerequisite. While a number of such algorithms have been presented in the past, an automatic thorough evaluation remains challenging. In that context, a new public database of ultrasound and MRI volumes acquired during glioma surgery [1] was made available, which includes multiple sets of anatomical landmark points to allow for Ground Truth matching. In the following, we present the results of our image-based registration algorithm on this data. The method is based on the multi-modal similarity metric denoted linear correlation of linear combinations, or LC^2 [2] and has recently been used in a first live evaluation during surgery [3]. Other popular approaches for image-based registration utilize gradient orientations [4], or self-similarity [5].

© Springer Nature Switzerland AG 2018
D. Stoyanov et al. (Eds.): POCUS 2018/BIVPCS 2018/CuRIOUS 2018/CPM 2018,
LNCS 11042, pp. 146–151, 2018.
https://doi.org/10.1007/978-3-030-01045-4_17

2   Method

In summary, the registration algorithm is based on optimizing a specific ultrasound-tailored multi-modal similarity metric denoted LC^2 on 3D patches of the MRI and ultrasound volumes. A non-linear optimization algorithm changes the values of a parametric transformation model to maximize it. While the LC^2 formulation is invariant with respect to modality-specific differences in appearance, it should be restricted to volume areas whose structures match when registered. Therefore it is advisable to remove the bright stripe on the skin surface of the ultrasound volumes, since it is missing in MRI. This would be trivial to do before ultrasound volume compounding; since the available data only has reconstructed volumes, a slightly more complex approach is necessary. The ultrasound volumes can have any orientation with respect to how the voxels are arranged in memory. Therefore we traverse the volumes along all axis both forward and reverse, and sum over occurrences of black, followed by intensities above a threshold for at least 1.5 mm. From the six directions, we choose the one with the most such occurrences and delete those skin sections with a 4 mm thickness. This cuts sufficient surface if the angle to the volume axis is oblique, and slightly more than necessary if it aligns with it.

The registration is implemented in the proprietary ImFusion SDK with full OpenGL-based GPU acceleration. The ultrasound volume is assigned as fixed volume, resampled to 0.5 mm (half the MRI voxel size), and properly zero-masked. The chosen similarity metric patch-size is 7^3 voxels, as optimized in prior work. Two non-linear optimizers successively operate on the parameters of a rigid pose from the initialization as provided by the navigation system. The first is a global DIRECT (DIviding RECTangles) sub-division method [6] searching on translation only, followed by a local BOBYQA (Bound Optimization BY Quadratic Approximation) algorithm [7] on all six parameters. Optionally, the local optimizer then executes another search on full affine parameters in order to accomodate non-uniform scaling and shearing of the data, or optimizes any other parametric transformation model. As an alternative to that, a dense-deformable Demons algorithm can create local forces based on the LC^2 patch values, iteratively updating and smoothing those forces until convergence. The average computation time is ≈ 20 s on a laptop with a NVIDIA GTX 1050 mobile GPU for the global and local rigid models, with an extra 10 s for the Demons algorithm if used. A dedicated workstation GPU is typically around 3–4 times faster, allowing for almost instant results during surgery after the ultrasound volumes have been acquired.

3   Evaluation

Table 1 shows our results, put alongside the best rigid and affine transformation that can be derived from the Ground Truth landmarks. In most of the cases, the error after rigid image-based registration is within a millimeter of the smallest rigid transformation that can be fit to the landmarks. The remaining ones

Table 1. Registration results in terms of residual landmark errors in mm.

Case	Landmarks			Image-based		
	Before	Rigid	Affine	Rigid	Affine	Demons
1	1.82	1.21	1.07	1.72	1.55	2.03
2	5.68	1.37	1.10	2.53	2.54	2.54
3	9.58	0.88	0.76	1.33	1.37	1.22
4	2.99	1.11	0.98	1.65	2.27	1.72
5	12.02	1.16	0.93	1.50	1.76	1.92
6	3.27	1.14	0.81	1.67	1.65	1.66
7	1.82	1.37	1.21	1.57	2.29	1.63
8	2.63	1.37	1.06	1.94	1.92	1.99
12	19.68	1.01	0.92	1.06	1.09	1.07
13	4.57	1.03	0.95	3.74	3.07	3.02
14	3.03	1.03	1.00	1.20	1.12	1.20
15	3.21	1.48	1.28	1.91	1.83	1.89
16	3.39	1.09	0.90	1.24	1.30	1.34
17	6.39	1.30	1.02	1.71	1.35	1.64
18	3.56	0.85	0.76	1.24	1.42	1.59
19	3.28	0.97	0.81	2.12	2.69	2.85
21	4.55	0.95	0.74	1.87	1.67	1.84
23	7.01	0.99	0.70	1.89	1.47	1.85
24	1.10	0.83	0.74	1.12	1.01	1.10
25	10.06	1.32	0.87	2.78	2.55	2.12
26	2.83	1.18	0.98	1.36	1.24	1.48
27	5.76	1.18	1.05	1.44	1.70	2.22
Mean	**5.37**	**1.13**	**0.94**	**1.75**	**1.77**	**1.81**

were visually inspected and all but one deemed well registered too; only case 13 exhibits an apparent slight rotation with respect to the Ground Truth (while still improving on the original landmark error before registration).

A more thorough accuracy evaluation is complicated by the fact that the landmarks themselves only have a limited accuracy. The residual errors denoted in the left columns of Table 1 are contributed to by two factors, namely (1) the localization error of experts selecting the point correspondences, and (2) the misfit of the rigid and affine transformation models on the given data. The average landmark error of ≈ 1 mm would hence be an upper bound for the localization error given a perfect rigid or affine registration. Most likely though, such a transformation model is not entirely sufficent even on the pre-resection data at hand due to tissue deformations, and possibly tracking and calibration errors.

To investigate further, we are using the hypothesis that both the landmark errors as well as the LC^2 similarity metric reveal the accuracy of the registration down to a certain scale. If they both improve (in a reciprocal way of course, since we are comparing error values to a similarity metric), the chosen transformation model most likely improved the alignment. Table 2 shows the LC^2 similarity measure values for the same transformation models as shown in the error table, with one addition: We use a parametric deformation similar to radial basis functions (RBF), where an inverse distance formulation is used to interpolate between the landmark locations in the most smooth possible way. Hence, the landmark error here is forced to zero up to a numerical epsilon due to the distance field inversion. However, as can be seen in the RBF column in the table, the LC^2 value for this model is slightly worse than the affine fit. This suggests that here, the deformation might be overfit to the point correspondences

Table 2. LC^2 similarity metric on all data for the different transformation models.

Case	Landmarks				Image-based		
	Before	Rigid	Affine	RBF	Rigid	Affine	Demons
1	0.157	0.174	0.179	0.174	0.183	0.192	0.196
2	0.145	0.179	0.174	0.194	0.195	0.195	0.215
3	0.167	0.239	0.246	0.233	0.245	0.268	0.276
4	0.169	0.188	0.191	0.194	0.196	0.230	0.222
5	0.182	0.248	0.255	0.246	0.265	0.297	0.317
6	0.164	0.184	0.187	0.184	0.200	0.216	0.213
7	0.138	0.144	0.150	0.145	0.147	0.166	0.168
8	0.203	0.231	0.239	0.233	0.247	0.273	0.291
12	0.149	0.269	0.276	0.266	0.271	0.296	0.309
13	0.174	0.190	0.203	0.192	0.227	0.229	0.245
14	0.162	0.230	0.235	0.227	0.240	0.242	0.258
15	0.163	0.184	0.189	0.187	0.194	0.194	0.221
16	0.191	0.245	0.245	0.253	0.253	0.271	0.285
17	0.177	0.247	0.255	0.253	0.258	0.282	0.289
18	0.186	0.229	0.221	0.235	0.258	0.273	0.279
19	0.195	0.232	0.230	0.227	0.240	0.265	0.270
21	0.149	0.175	0.178	0.173	0.201	0.207	0.225
23	0.172	0.240	0.252	0.260	0.252	0.264	0.278
24	0.192	0.204	0.208	0.202	0.209	0.215	0.205
25	0.136	0.173	0.199	0.177	0.170	0.179	0.187
26	0.217	0.276	0.298	0.278	0.287	0.308	0.312
27	0.153	0.198	0.199	0.203	0.203	0.242	0.227
Mean	**0.170**	**0.213**	**0.218**	**0.215**	**0.225**	**0.241**	**0.250**

including their localization errors as opposed to actual structural deformations. It is also illustrated by the example in Fig. 1(b). Apart from that, the similarity consistently increases from the initial transformation, over rigid, to affine. Likewise, it increases for the image-based rigid and affine model with the highest improvement on the dense demons model. Most notably, the similarity improvements are each significantly higher than the corresponding change in landmark errors in Table 1, again suggesting a better alignment towards the right columns.

In terms of a statistical analysis, in Table 1 the only columns that are not significantly different are the various image-based transformation models (three right-most columns, Rigid/Affine/Demons), i.e. the landmark errors are all in the same order of magnitude. In Table 2, columns 2–4 (landmarks rigid vs. RBF), 3–4 (landmarks affine vs. RBF) and 3–5 (landmarks affine vs. image-based rigid) are insignificantly different. A paired Wilcoxon test with a p-value threshold of 0.01 was used. All other results are significantly different, hence it is obvious that registering landmarks only versus using our image-based method produces different results, each favoring their metric.

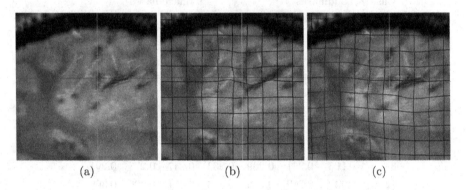

(a)   (b)   (c)

Fig. 1. Registration on case 1, **(a)** rigid with our method, **(b)** RBF on landmarks, **(c)** Demons with our method.

4   Conclusion

We have presented an algorithm for fully automatic registration of pre-resection ultrasound to pre-operative MRI volumes during brain surgery, which improves the registration for all 22 cases. For the majority of cases, the used transformation models yield landmark errors only slightly worse than the best landmark fit (in the order of magnitude of the localization errors). Since it is also known that the fiducial registration errors (here on the provided landmarks) cannot be used to reliably predict the error of a clinical target such as the tumor center [8], further validation should be performed on Ground Truth segmentations of the actual tumor mass, e.g. by computing Dice overlap values.

It will certainly also be quite interesting to locally compare regions where the LC^2 similarity metric causes a systematic shift away from the true alignment, because the local linearity assumptions are violated by the complex underlying imaging physics. Such occurrences could be improved upon with Deep Learning techniques, either by (1) learning a weighting of how reliable the similarity metric is, or (2) directly learning a more non-linear version of the similarity metric that is also taking more image content than its own patch into account.

Regarding the transformation model, it is apparent that the pre-resection data is mostly but not entirely rigid; here, a custom parametric model could be developed, for example using parameter reduction techniques on all available landmarks, also taking the position of the ultrasound probe into account where compression is strongest. To eventually achieve higher clinical impact, techniques should be developed to also continuously register ultrasound volumes during and after resection and always visualize information from the pre-operative plan accordingly. Besides a more elaborate transformation model, this will also require to exclude the resection site from registration, since it only has been changed in one of the images.

Acknowledgments. Thanks to the entire team at ImFusion, both for some additional software development supporting this work, as well as providing valuable feedback.

References

1. Xiao, Y., Fortin, M., Unsgård, G., Rivaz, H., Reinertsen, I.: Retrospective evaluation of cerebral tumors (RESECT): a clinical database of pre-operative MRI and intra-operative ultrasound in low-grade glioma surgeries. Med. Phys. **44**, 3875–3882 (2017)
2. Wein, W., Ladikos, A., Fuerst, B., Shah, A., Sharma, K., Navab, N.: Global registration of ultrasound to MRI using the LC^2 metric for enabling neurosurgical guidance. In: Mori, K., Sakuma, I., Sato, Y., Barillot, C., Navab, N. (eds.) MICCAI 2013. LNCS, vol. 8149, pp. 34–41. Springer, Heidelberg (2013). https://doi.org/10.1007/978-3-642-40811-3_5
3. Reinertsen, I., Iversen, D., Lindseth, F., Wein, W., Unsgård, G.: Intra-operative ultrasound based correction of brain-shift. In: Intraoperative Imaging Society Conference, Hanover, Germany (2017)
4. De Nigris, D., Collins, L., Arbel, T.: Fast rigid registration of pre-operative magnetic resonance images to intra-operative ultrasound for neurosurgery based on high confidence gradient orientations. Int. J. Comput. Assist. Radiol. Surg. **8**, 649–661 (2013)
5. Heinrich, M., et al.: MIND: modality independent neighbourhood descriptor for multi-modal deformable registration. Med. Image Anal. **16**, 1423–1435 (2012)
6. Jones, D., Perttunen, C., Stuckmann, B.: Lipschitzian optimization without the lipschitz constant. J. Optim. Theory Appl. **79**, 157 (1993)
7. Powell, M.J.: The BOBYQA Algorithm for Bound Constrained Optimization without Derivatives. Cambridge Report NA2009/06, University of Cambridge (2009)
8. Fitzpatrick, J.: Fiducial registration error and target registration error are uncorrelated. In: Miga, M., Wong, I., Kenneth, H. (eds.) Proceedings of the SPIE, vol. 7261 (2009)

Deformable MRI-Ultrasound Registration Using 3D Convolutional Neural Network

Li Sun[✉] and Songtao Zhang

Southern University of Science and Technology, Shenzhen 518055, China
lisun97@foxmail.com

Abstract. Precise tracking of intra-operative tissue shift is important for accurate resection of brain tumor. Alignment of pre-interventional magnetic resonance imaging (MRI) to intra-operative ultrasound (iUS) is required to access tissue shift and enable guided surgery. However, accurate and robust image registration needed to relate pre-interventional MRI to iUS images is difficult due to the very different nature of image intensity between modalities. Here we present a framework that can perform non-rigid MRI-ultrasound registration using 3D convolutional neural network (CNN). The framework is composed of three components: feature extractor, deformation field generator and spatial sampler. Our automatic registration framework adopts unsupervised learning approach, allows accurate end-to-end deformable MRI-ultrasound registration. Our proposed method avoids the downfall of intensity-based methods by considering both image intensity and gradient. It achieves competitive registration accuracy on RESECT dataset. In addition, our method takes only about one second to register each image pair, enabling applications such as real time registration.

Keywords: MRI-ultrasound registration · 3D CNN · Deep learning

1 Introduction

Radiological imaging is commonly used for diagnosis, treatment and scientific research. Different modalities of techniques are often used concordantly in practice because they complement with each other. MRI measures the relaxation times of the ^{1}H nuclei, it can provide visualization for the overall structure and anatomy, while iUS measures the changes in acoustic impedance, it is relative inexpensive and allows for intra-operative detection.

Image registration refers to the spatial alignment of images into the same coordinate system. It can greatly facilitate a wide range of medical applications from diagnosis to therapy. As far as brain tumor resection is concerned, accurate registration can provide the boundary of brain tumor and corresponding tissue shift. Many algorithms and software toolkits have been developed for image registration [1,5]. However, most current methods focus on registration within

© Springer Nature Switzerland AG 2018
D. Stoyanov et al. (Eds.): POCUS 2018/BIVPCS 2018/CuRIOUS 2018/CPM 2018,
LNCS 11042, pp. 152–158, 2018.
https://doi.org/10.1007/978-3-030-01045-4_18

modality and are based on intensity values. These intensity-based registration methods may fail in inter-modality registration tasks, such as MRI-iUS image registration. This is due to the different underlying principles of imaging techniques and striking difference in field of views. Inter-modality image registration poses special challenges and robust and accurate methods are still desired.

In recent years, deep convolutional neural networks (CNNs) have achieved great success in the field of computer vision. Inspired by the biological structure of visual cortex, CNNs are artificial neural networks with multiple hidden convolutional layers between the input and output layers. They have non-linear property and are capable of extracting higher level representative features. CNNs have been applied into a wide range of fields and achieved state-of-the-art performance on tasks such as image recognition, instance detection, and semantic segmentation. In this paper, we propose a novel learning-based framework for MRI-iUS image registration. It is composed of three parts: feature extractor, deformation field generator and spatial sampler. Our automatic registration framework allows accurate and fast MRI-ultrasound registration.

2   Related Work

2.1   Intensity-Based Approaches for Registration

To date, a lot of traditional intensity-based methods have been reported for medical image registration [1,5]. These methods usually include the following steps. First, a transformation model is selected to deform the moving image and spatially align the intensity between fixed image and deformed moving image. The choice of transformation model depends on the complexity of deformations required. For example, simple transformation such as rigid, affine and B-spline transformation are enough to recover underlying rigid deformations. In more complicated cases, more flexible non-parametric transformation models are used to recover complex deformations.

Second, a similarity metric is defined to how well two images are matched after transformation. The selection of the similarity metric, also called the cost function, depends on the intrinsic properties of images to be registered and deformation complexity. Commonly used metrics include sum of squared distances, normalized cross-correlation (NCC), mutual information (MI) and others.

Finally, iterative optimization method is applied to update the transformation parameters to minimize the cost function. Traditional medical image registration methods have achieved acceptable result in many registration tasks. But there are two downfalls for these methods. First, most of methods focus on aligning image intensity, which may fail in inter-modality image registration. For example, MRI and iUS image have strikingly different fields of view, which is due to different nature in imaging principles. In addition, minimizing cost function by iterative optimization is slow, which may hinder application of image registration.

2.2 Learning-Based Approaches for Registration

Several studies have exploited learning-based approaches for image registration [6,8]. Recently, CNNs have been applied to many computer vision tasks, including image registration. Deep CNNs contain many hidden layers so that they can non-linearly transform input data and extract higher level features, thus by training it can learn to determine the optimal decision boundary in the high-dimensional feature space. Wu et al. [8] utilize convolutional stacked auto-encoder to select deep feature representations in image patches, then estimate the deformation pathway. Miao et al. [6] use convolutional neural network to predict a transformation matrix, which is then used to perform rigid registration. In this paper, we follow these ideas and propose an end-to-end model for deformable image registration in an unsupervised learning way.

2.3 Spatial Transformer Network (STN)

Jaderberg et al. [4] proposed the spatial transformer network, which enables the learning of spatial transformation. STN is a fully differentiable module so that it can be inserted into existing convolutional neural networks, giving CNNs the ability to spatially transform feature maps. STN takes transformation parameters as input, then it generates a sampling grid according to the parameters. The sampling grid is used to spatially transform image by bilinear interpolation. By training with supervision, STN is capable to learn a dynamic mechanism to actively spatially transform an image by producing an appropriate transformation for each input voxel, including scaling, cropping, rotations, as well as non-rigid deformations. de Vos et al. [7] applied STN to handwritten digit registration, but it requires large amount of data for training.

3 Methodology

3.1 Problem Statement

In image registration, the moving image I_M, is deformed to match the corresponding image I_F called the fixed image. Thus, the deformed image $\tilde{I}$ can be expressed as

$$\tilde{I} = I_M(x + u(x)) \tag{1}$$

where x denotes a three-dimensional coordinate and u represents the deformation field. In this work, we attempt to predict the optimal deformation field $u(x)$ to register MRI to corresponding iUS image.

3.2   Registration Framework

Our registration framework is composed of three components: feature extractor, deformation field generator and spatial sampler. The overall workflow is illustrated in Fig. 1:

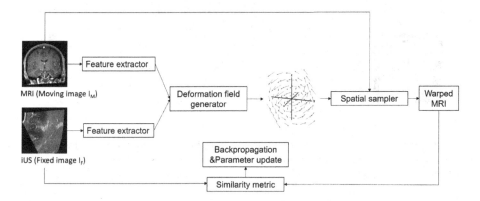

Fig. 1. Framework overview

For feature extractor, two fully convolutional neural networks are used to extract higher level representative features from MRI and iUS images respectively. Each network contains three convolutional layers with 16 kernels sized $3 \times 3 \times 3$, coupled with batch normalization and exponential linear units for activation. The extracted features are concatenated and fed into the deformation field generator.

The deformation field generator takes features extracted from both MRI and iUS images as input, and it produces a deformation field as output. The structure of deformation field generator is inspired by FlowNet [2], which is original used to estimate optic flow. It is composed of a contracting part and an expanding part. The contracting part includes three convolutional layers and a downsampling layer, which is used to capture context and deep level features. The expanding part is consisted of a upsampling layer and three convolutional layers, which is used to restore details and produce a deformation field the same size as the input image. Skip connections are also incorporated to integrate both high-level and low-level features. All layers contain 16 filters sized $3 \times 3 \times 3$, and are coupled with batch normalization and exponential linear units for activation, except for the last layer which use linear activation. The resulting deformation field is fed into the spatial sampler (Fig. 2).

Finally, a spatial sampler is used to apply the deformation field to regular spatial grid, resulting in the sampling grid. The MRI image is resampled by bilinear interpolation. And the deformed MRI image is aligned to the iUS image to calculate the similarity. The loss is backpropagated into the network and update the parameters. The training process is unsupervised as it does not need expert-labeled landmark data.

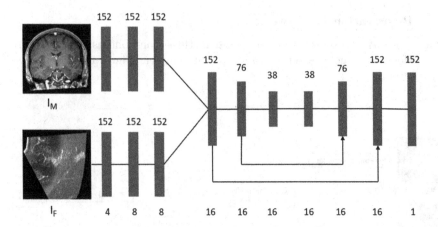

Fig. 2. Detailed structures of feature extractor and deformation field generator. Note that the size and number of channels of each feature map are shown on the top and bottom of figure respectively.

3.3   Similarity Metric

We evaluate the registration quality by considering both the image intensity and gradient. Many conventional intensity-based methods are not appropriate for this inter-modality registration task, because MRI and iUS images have very different nature in intensity values. To tackle this, we assume that the US intensity value $u_i = I_M(x + u(x))$ for voxel i is either correlated with the corresponding MRI intensity value or with the MRI image gradient magnitude $g_i = |\nabla p_i|$. As suggested by Fuerst et al. [3] that, ultrasound intensity values may describe different properties of internal fluids and tissues as well as represent tissue interfaces or gradients. Thus, we define the loss function as:

$$\sum_{x \in \phi} (I_F(x) - (\alpha p_i + \beta g_i + \gamma))^2 \tag{2}$$

in which α, β and γ are learnt parameters during training. We assume that the network will automatically find the optimal parameter to make the deformed MRI image best fit with the iUS image.

4   Experiments

4.1   Dataset

We use the publicly available RESECT dataset [9] for training and validation. The dataset provides pre-operative T1w and T2-FLAIR MRI and iUS images from 23 patients. It also provides expert-labeled homologous anatomical landmarks, defined on all image modalities. All data were acquired for routine clinical care at St Olavs University Hospital, after patients gave their informed consent. The imaging data are available in both MINC and NIFTI formats.

4.2   Preprocessing

We use T1w MRI scans and before resection intra-operative US images for training and validation, which account for 22 image pairs. We split 18 cases for training phase and 4 cases for validation phase. We downsample all images to $150 \times 150 \times 150$ to reduce memory usage and suppress speckle noise. In order to augment the training data, we applied random flipping, rotation, cropping, as well as random gaussian noise to the images.

4.3   Result

In order to evaluate the performance of our method, we applied the trained model on validation dataset and calculated the mean target registration errors (mTREs) between the predicted landmark positions on the iUS images and ground truth. The evaluation results in training phase and validation phase are listed as follows (Table 1):

Table 1. Evaluation result

Phase	mTREs (mm)	Std. (mm)	Process time per image (sec)
Training	4.73	2.71	2.66
Validation	3.91	0.53	1.21

4.4   Implementation Details

To implement the algorithm, we use Tensorflow framework and a NVIDIA Tesla M40 GPU accelerator. We use stochastic gradient descent optimizer with momentum 0.9, and set initial learning rate to 0.001. We also set the number of epoch for training 20 and batch size to 3 for training.

5   Conclusion

In this paper, we present a framework that can perform non-rigid MRI-ultrasound registration using 3D convolutional neural network. This framework is composed of feature extractor, deformation field generator and spatial sampler. Our fully automatic registration framework adopts a learning-based approach and it avoids the downfall of intensity-based methods by considering both image intensity and gradient. In addition, our method only takes one second to register each image pair. Moreover, our method is unsupervised, without the requirement for expert-curated landmarks for training. The evaluation result on RESECT dataset demonstrated that our proposed method achieves competitive registration accuracy, and it can be applied to other cross-modality image registration tasks. In the future, we will explore more possibilities of optimizing network structure and penalizing shadow regions as suggested by Fuerst et al. [3].

References

1. Avants, B.B., Tustison, N., Song, G.: Advanced Normalization Tools (ANTs). Insight J. **2**, 1–35 (2009)
2. Dosovitskiy, A., et al.: FlowNet: learning optical flow with convolutional networks. In: Proceedings of the IEEE International Conference on Computer Vision, pp. 2758–2766 (2015)
3. Fuerst, B., Wein, W., Müller, M., Navab, N.: Automatic ultrasound-MRI registration for neurosurgery using the 2D and 3D LC^2 metric. Med. Image Anal. **18**(8), 1312–1319 (2014)
4. Jaderberg, M., Simonyan, K., Zisserman, A., et al.: Spatial transformer networks. In: Advances in Neural Information Processing Systems, pp. 2017–2025 (2015)
5. Klein, S., Staring, M., Murphy, K., Viergever, M.A., Pluim, J.P.: Elastix: a toolbox for intensity-based medical image registration. IEEE Trans. Med. Imaging **29**(1), 196–205 (2010)
6. Miao, S., Wang, Z.J., Zheng, Y., Liao, R.: Real-time 2D/3D registration via CNN regression. In: 2016 IEEE 13th International Symposium on Biomedical Imaging (ISBI), pp. 1430–1434. IEEE (2016)
7. de Vos, B.D., Berendsen, F.F., Viergever, M.A., Staring, M., Išgum, I.: End-to-end unsupervised deformable image registration with a convolutional neural network. In: Cardoso, M.J. (ed.) DLMIA/ML-CDS -2017. LNCS, vol. 10553, pp. 204–212. Springer, Cham (2017). https://doi.org/10.1007/978-3-319-67558-9_24
8. Wu, G., Kim, M., Wang, Q., Munsell, B.C., Shen, D.: Scalable high-performance image registration framework by unsupervised deep feature representations learning. IEEE Trans. Biomed. Eng. **63**(7), 1505–1516 (2016)
9. Xiao, Y., Fortin, M., Unsgård, G., Rivaz, H., Reinertsen, I.: REtroSpective Evaluation of Cerebral Tumors (RESECT): a clinical database of pre-operative MRI and intra-operative ultrasound in low-grade glioma surgeries. Med. Phys. **44**(7), 3875–3882 (2017)

Intra-operative Ultrasound to MRI Fusion with a Public Multimodal Discrete Registration Tool

Mattias P. Heinrich[✉]

Institute of Medical Informatics, University of Lübeck, Lübeck, Germany
heinrich@imi.uni-luebeck.de
http://www.mpheinrich.de/

Abstract. We present accurate results for multi-modal fusion of intra-operative 3D ultrasound and magnetic resonance imaging (MRI) using the publicly available and robust discrete registration approach *deeds*. After pre-processing the scans to have isotropic voxel sizes of 0.5 mm and a common coordinate system, we run both linear and deformable registration using the self-similarity context metric. We use default parameters that have previously been applied for multi-atlas fusion demonstrating the generalisation of the approach. Transformed landmark locations are obtained by either directly applying the nonlinear warp or fitting a rigid transform with six parameters. The two approaches yield average target registration errors of 1.88 mm and 1.67 mm respectively on the 22 training scans of the CuRIOUS challenge. Optimising the regularisation weight can further improve this to 1.62 mm (within 0.5 mm of the theoretical lower bound). Our findings demonstrate that in contrast to classification and segmentation tasks, multimodal registration can be appropriately handled without designing domain-specific algorithms and without any expert supervision.

1 Introduction and Related Work

Fusion of multimodal medical data is one of the most important application of image registration. In radiotherapy the registration of a computed tomography (CT) scan for dose-planning and an MRI for tumour and organs-at-risk delineation have to be aligned in a nonlinear fashion. In ultrasound guided neurosurgery an intra-operative 3D ultrasound (3DUS) has to be registered to a pre-treatment MRI to guide the surgeon during tumour resection. The correction of challenge on brainshift in intra-operative ultrasound (CuRIOUS) addresses the latter and provides a large training dataset of 22 clinical multimodal cases of 3T MRI T1w and T2 FLAIR scans as well as 3DUS after craniotomy but before dura opening with expert-labeled homologous anatomical landmarks as presented and described in detail in [1]. The main challenges that were discussed in previous

© Springer Nature Switzerland AG 2018
D. Stoyanov et al. (Eds.): POCUS 2018/BIVPCS 2018/CuRIOUS 2018/CPM 2018,
LNCS 11042, pp. 159–164, 2018.
https://doi.org/10.1007/978-3-030-01045-4_19

work revolve around a suitable way to define modality-invariant similarity metrics and fast and robust algorithm for finding the transform that optimises this measure. Popular choices of metrics for MRI-US registration include gradient-based correlation metrics [2], self-similarity descriptors [3] or advanced mutual information variants [4]. Secondly, a suitable optimisation framework has to be adapted to enable optimal performance on the given dataset. In this submission, we argue that excellent results can be achieved by employing off-the-shelf and publicly available algorithms that have been optimised for general medical image registration tasks, such as atlas-based segmentation propagation of abdominal CT, without any further domain specific adaption. In the next section, we will describe the employed method that is based on self-similarity context (SSC) descriptors [3] and the discrete optimisation framework *deeds* [5] that performed best in two MICCAI segmentation challenges Beyond the Cranial Vault (BVC) in 2015 [6] and Multimodal Whole-Heart Segmentation (MM-WHS) in 2017 [7] with the exact same default parameters and a subsequent label fusion step.

2   Method

Quantised **self-similarity context** descriptors (SSC) [3] are used to define a similarity metric. Instead of relying on direct intensity comparisons across scans, SSC aims to extract modality-invariant neighbourhood representations separately within each scan based on local self-similarities (normalised patch-distances). It naturally deals well with multi-modal alignment problems, enables contrast invariance, which is particularly beneficial for MRI scans, and focuses the alignment on image edges of the ultrasound.

The **dense displacement sampling** registration short *deeds* [5] is a discrete optimisation algorithm that aims to avoid local minima in the cost function. It is therefore in particular suitable for challenging image appearance often seen in intra-operative ultrasound. A dense displacement sampling covers a large range of potential displacements (capture range) and the combinatorial optimisation based on dynamic programming ensures plausible first-order B-spline transformations without unrealistic deformations on a specified control-point grid. A diffusion regularisation is used between edges that connect neighbouring displacement nodes and this graph is simplified to contain no loops (a minimum-spanning-tree) to simplify the optimisation. A symmetry constraint on the non-linear transform further increases the smoothness of deformations.

3   Implementation

We used *c3d*, which is a general purpose medical image processing command-line tool and can be found at http://www.itksnap.org/pmwiki/pmwiki.php?n=Downloads.C3D to resample the provided nifti files of 3DUS and T2 FLAIR into a common reference frame and to isotropic voxel sizes of $0.5\,\mathrm{mm}^3$. The command used for the MRI FLAIR and 3DUS data respectively therefore was:

```
c3d *folder*/Case1-US-before.nii.gz *folder*/Case1-FLAIR.nii.gz
  -reslice-identity -resample-mm 0.5x0.5x0.5mm -o Case1-MRI_in_US.nii.gz
c3d *folder*/Case1-US-before.nii.gz -resample-mm 0.5x0.5x0.5mm -o Case1-US.nii.gz
```

We then used both linear and deformable parts of the *deeds* framework as downloaded from https://github.com/mattiaspaul/deedsBCV/ with default settings. These include an linear pre-registration that performs a block-matching on four scale levels and estimates a rigid transformation using:

```
linearBCV -F Case1-US.nii.gz -M Case1-MRI_in_US.nii.gz -R 1 -O affine1
```

In order to be able to apply the estimated linear and nonlinear transformations to manual landmark positions, the algorithm requires segmentation masks. In our case, these will represent landmarks as 3D spheres. After generating two text files with a custom python implementation[1]. The landmark segmentations can be easily generated using *c3d* as follows:

```
python landmarks_split_txt.py --inputtag *folder*/Case1-MRI-beforeUS.tag --savetxt Case1_lm
c3d Case1-MRI_in_US.nii.gz -scale 0 -landmarks-to-spheres Case1_lm_mri.txt 1
  -o Case1-MRI-landmarks.nii.gz
```

The transformation matrix is fed into the deformable part of *deeds* using the following (default) parameters: number of displacement steps $l_{\max} = [8, 7, 6, 5, 4]$, quantisation/stride $q = [5, 4, 3, 2, 1]$, and B-spline grid spacings of $[8, 7, 6, 5, 4]$ voxels. A default weighting of $\alpha = 1.6$ between the SSC-similarity and the diffusion regularisation in *deeds* was used. An example command to run a registration is as follows:

```
deedsBCV -F Case1-MRI_in_US.nii.gz -M Case1-US.nii.gz -O Case1-deeds
  -S Case1-US-landmarks.nii.gz -A affine1_matrix.txt
```

The computation times are approx. $5\,\mathrm{s}$ for linear alignment and $20\,\mathrm{s}$ for deformable registration on a mobile dual-core CPU based on the efficient OpenMP implementation.

After applying the combined transformations to the 3D landmark spheres, their spatial (voxel) coordinates are extracted by calculating the centre of mass in python using[2] and the following command, which stores them in a text file and can directly calculate the mTRE when provided with the target landmarks:

```
python landmarks_centre_mass.py --inputnii Case1-MRI-landmarks.nii.gz
  --movingnii Case1-deeds_deformed_seg.nii.gz --savetxt Case1-results
```

In the next sections the results are presented both visually and numerically and their implications are discussed.

4   Results and Discussion

All experiments were run with same settings on the 22 training scans of the challenge and evaluated using all manual landmarks as provided by the organisers. The algorithms are fully automatic and require no manual initialisation.

---

[1] https://gist.github.com/mattiaspaul/56a49fa792ef6f143e56699a06067712.
[2] https://gist.github.com/mattiaspaul/f4183f525b1cbc65e71ad23298d6436e.

Table 1. Numerical results of accuracy of multimodal registration evaluated with manual landmarks in mm using the *deeds* algorithm in three different settings. First, only the linear part is considered, which yields an mTRE of 1.88 ± 0.53 mm. Second, a nonlinear transform is estimated in addition, yielding a slightly higher error of 1.92 ± 0.60 mm. But when finally fitting another rigid transform to the nonlinear result, the best mTRE of 1.67 ± 0.54 mm is reached.

Case	#1	#2	#3	#4	#5	#6	#7	#8	#12	#13	#14	stddev
Before	1.86	5.75	9.63	2.98	12.20	3.34	1.88	2.65	19.76	4.71	3.03	4.29
Linear	1.88	2.38	1.29	1.31	1.87	1.86	1.58	2.66	1.43	3.47	1.33	0.53
Nonlinear	2.60	2.58	2.29	1.35	2.12	2.30	1.63	2.95	1.21	1.70	1.91	0.60
NL+fit	1.45	2.21	2.00	1.20	1.64	1.89	1.46	3.22	1.14	1.18	1.18	0.54
Case	#15	#16	#17	#18	#19	#21	#23	#24	#25	#26	#27	**avg**
Before	3.37	3.41	6.41	3.66	3.16	4.46	7.05	1.13	10.10	2.93	5.86	**5.42**
Linear	2.32	1.41	1.78	1.23	2.12	1.90	1.59	1.57	3.21	1.60	1.58	**1.88**
Nonlinear	1.97	1.73	2.20	1.27	2.29	1.50	1.33	2.54	1.29	1.23	2.30	**1.92**
NL+fit	1.89	1.50	1.78	1.03	2.05	1.30	1.21	2.69	1.45	1.31	1.86	**1.67**

We confirmed that the original error (before registration) was approx. 5.4 mm as mentioned in [1]. The numerical results are presented in Table 1 and using distribution plots in Fig. 2. A clear advantage over the initial error can be seen from 5.42 mm to 1.88 mm when using a linear transform only. We were also interested in exploring whether the nonlinear part of the registration may provide a better alignment despite the fact that the ultrasound images were acquired

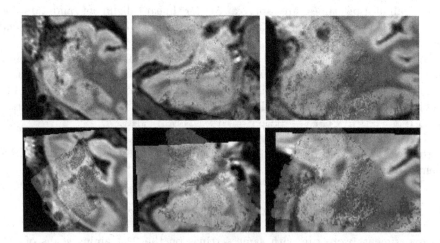

Fig. 1. Visual example of US-MRI registration for #3 of the training dataset. The top row shows a colour overlay (US in jet) on top of the original MRI. The bottom row demonstrates a clearly improved alignment when applying the automatically estimated linear transform to the MRI scan.

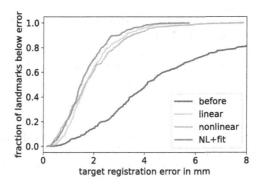

Fig. 2. Cumulative distribution of landmark errors sorted in ascending order. All variants of the automated multimodal discrete registration decrease the landmark error and improve image alignment.

before opening the dura. This is not directly the case as the result slightly deteriorate to 1.92 mm on average. However, when fitting again a rigid transform to the nonlinearly displaced landmark correspondences a mTRE of 1.67 mm. The fitting has been carried out using the technique described in [8]. This indicates that the more flexible deformable registration can improve the match of certain landmarks, but is also less robust in areas of limited contrast. Therefore, the following restriction to a rigid transform, which reduces the influence of outliers, improves the overall outcome.

We further noted that aligning MRI to ultrasound is slightly more accurate than in reverse order. Since, the nonlinear part of *deeds* is already symmetric this discrepancy could be alleviated by using the approach of [9]. Furthermore, the regularisation parameter could be further optimised from $\alpha = 1.6$ to $\alpha = 0.4$ yielding a modest improvement to 1.62 mm mTRE. A visual example of the registration and multi-modal fusion outcome is shown in Fig. 1.

5 Conclusion and Outlook

In summary, we have demonstrated that the general purpose, publicly available, discrete registration toolbox *deeds* provides excellent accuracies of 1.62 mm for a challenging ultrasound to MRI brain registration. The method relies on no training data, but potentially the widely applicable self-similarity descriptors could be replaced by a learning-based approach that relies on known correspondences cf. [10] or [11]. However, the impact will probably be more pronounced when considering scans with more brain-shift.

A further interesting research direction would be to only learn the spatial layout used for self-similarity distance computations by means of deformable convolutions. These have been successfully applied to registration and segmentation tasks with few labelled datasets [12]. Moreover, the computation time of the algorithm could be drastically reduced (to subsecond runtimes) by performing the similarity and regularisation calculations on a GPU, which we have already demonstrated for parts of the algorithm in [13] and we intend to complete this for the whole algorithm in the near future.

Acknowledgements. We would like to thank the CuRIOUS 2018 organisers for providing this new multimodal dataset to the public.

References

1. Xiao, Y., Fortin, M., Unsgård, G., Rivaz, H., Reinertsen, I.: Retrospective evaluation of cerebral tumors (RESECT): a clinical database of pre-operative MRI and intra-operative ultrasound in low-grade glioma surgeries. Med. Phys. **44**(7), 3875–3882 (2017)
2. Fuerst, B., Wein, W., Müller, M., Navab, N.: Automatic ultrasound-MRI registration for neurosurgery using the 2D and 3D LC2 metric. Med. Image Anal. **18**(8), 1312–1319 (2014)
3. Heinrich, M.P., Jenkinson, M., Papież, B.W., Brady, S.M., Schnabel, J.A.: Towards realtime multimodal fusion for image-guided interventions using self-similarities. In: Mori, K., Sakuma, I., Sato, Y., Barillot, C., Navab, N. (eds.) MICCAI 2013. LNCS, vol. 8149, pp. 187–194. Springer, Heidelberg (2013). https://doi.org/10.1007/978-3-642-40811-3_24
4. Rivaz, H., Karimaghaloo, Z., Collins, D.L.: Self-similarity weighted mutual information: a new nonrigid image registration metric. Med. Image Anal. **18**(2), 343–358 (2014)
5. Heinrich, M., Jenkinson, M., Brady, M., Schnabel, J.: MRF-based deformable registration and ventilation estimation of lung CT. IEEE Trans. Med. Imag. **32**(7), 1239–1248 (2013)
6. Xu, Z., et al.: Evaluation of six registration methods for the human abdomen on clinically acquired CT. IEEE Trans. Biomed. Eng. **63**(8), 1563–1572 (2016)
7. Heinrich, M.P., Oster, J.: MRI whole heart segmentation using discrete nonlinear registration and fast non-local fusion. In: Pop, M. (ed.) STACOM 2017. LNCS, vol. 10663, pp. 233–241. Springer, Cham (2018). https://doi.org/10.1007/978-3-319-75541-0_25
8. Arun, K.S., Huang, T.S., Blostein, S.D.: Least-squares fitting of two 3-D point sets. IEEE Trans. Pattern Anal. Mach. Intell. **5**, 698–700 (1987)
9. Modat, M., Cash, D.M., Daga, P., Winston, G.P., Duncan, J.S., Ourselin, S.: Global image registration using a symmetric block-matching approach. J. Med. Imaging **1**(2), 024003 (2014)
10. Masci, J., Bronstein, M.M., Bronstein, A.M., Schmidhuber, J.: Multimodal similarity-preserving hashing. IEEE Trans. Pattern Anal. Mach. Intell. **36**(4), 824–830 (2014)
11. Blendowski, M., Heinrich, M.P.: 3D-CNNs for deep binary descriptor learning in medical volume data. In: Maier, A., Deserno, T., Handels, H., Maier-Hein, K., Palm, C., Tolxdorff, T. (eds.) Bildverarbeitung für die Medizin 2018. I, pp. 23–28. Springer, Heidelberg (2018). https://doi.org/10.1007/978-3-662-56537-7_19
12. Heinrich, M.P., Oktay, O., Bouteldja, N.: OBELISK - one kernel to solve nearly everything: unified 3D binary convolutions for image analysis. In: Medical Imaging with Deep Learning (2018)
13. Ha, I.Y., Wilms, M., Handels, H., Heinrich, M.: Model-based sparse-to-dense image registration for realtime respiratory motion estimation in image-guided interventions. IEEE Trans. Biomed. Eng. (2018). https://doi.org/10.1109/TBME.2018.2837387

Deformable MRI-Ultrasound Registration via Attribute Matching and Mutual-Saliency Weighting for Image-Guided Neurosurgery

Inês Machado[1,2(✉)], Matthew Toews[3], Jie Luo[1,4], Prashin Unadkat[5],
Walid Essayed[5], Elizabeth George[1], Pedro Teodoro[2],
Herculano Carvalho[6], Jorge Martins[2], Polina Golland[7],
Steve Pieper[1,8], Sarah Frisken[1], Alexandra Golby[5],
William Wells III[1,7], and Yangming Ou[9]

[1] Department of Radiology, Brigham and Women's Hospital,
Harvard Medical School, Boston, MA, USA
[2] Instituto Superior Técnico, Universidade de Lisboa, Lisbon, Portugal
ines7.prata.machado@gmail.com
[3] École de Technologie Supérieure, Montreal, Canada
[4] Graduate School of Frontier Sciences, University of Tokyo, Tokyo, Japan
[5] Department of Neurosurgery, Brigham and Women's Hospital,
Harvard Medical School, Boston, MA, USA
[6] Department of Neurosurgery, Hospital de Santa Maria, CHLN,
Lisbon, Portugal
[7] Computer Science and Artificial Intelligence Laboratory, MIT,
Cambridge, MA, USA
[8] Isomics, Inc., Cambridge, MA, USA
[9] Department of Pediatrics and Radiology, Boston Children's Hospital,
Harvard Medical School, Boston, MA, USA

Abstract. Intraoperative brain deformation reduces the effectiveness of using preoperative images for intraoperative surgical guidance. We propose an algorithm for deformable registration of intraoperative ultrasound (US) and preoperative magnetic resonance (MR) images in the context of brain tumor resection. From each image voxel, a set of multi-scale and multi-orientation Gabor attributes is extracted from which optimal components are selected to establish a distinctive morphological signature of the anatomical and geometric context of its surroundings. To match the attributes across image pairs, we assign higher weights – higher mutual-saliency values - to those voxels more likely to establish reliable correspondences across images. The correlation coefficient is used as the similarity measure to evaluate effectiveness of the algorithm for multi-modal registration. Free-form deformation and discrete optimization are chosen as the deformation model and optimization strategy, respectively. Experiments demonstrate our methodology on registering preoperative T2-FLAIR MR to intraoperative US in 22 clinical cases. Using manually labelled corresponding landmarks between preoperative MR and intraoperative US images, we show that the mean target registration error decreases from an initial value of 5.37 ± 4.27 mm to 3.35 ± 1.19 mm after registration.

© Springer Nature Switzerland AG 2018
D. Stoyanov et al. (Eds.): POCUS 2018/BIVPCS 2018/CuRIOUS 2018/CPM 2018,
LNCS 11042, pp. 165–171, 2018.
https://doi.org/10.1007/978-3-030-01045-4_20

Keywords: Brain shift · Intraoperative ultrasound · Image registration
Attribute matching · Gabor filter bank · Mutual-saliency

1 Introduction

Brain shift combined with registration and tracking errors reduces the accuracy of image-guided neurosurgery based on neuronavigation systems [1–3]. Intraoperative ultrasound, being a real-time imaging modality, has the potential to enable the surgeon to accurately localize the instrument trajectories in the operative field and thus facilitate accurate resection to promote better surgical outcomes. However, registration of intraoperative US with preoperative MR images is a challenging problem due to the different information captured by each image modality. We present a deformable MR-US registration algorithm that uses attribute matching and mutual-saliency weighting and apply it to image-guided neurosurgery.

2 Methods

A registration framework usually consists of three parts: (1) the similarity measure, which defines the criterion to align the two images; (2) the deformation model, which defines the mechanism to transform one image to the other; and (3) the optimization strategy, which is used to determine the best parameters of the deformation model. An open question is how to define the similarity measure for MR-US registration. A deformable registration algorithm known as DRAMMS [4] has shown promise in defining similarity based on optimal Gabor attributes modulated by quantified matching reliabilities. It shows potential in handling large deformations and missing correspondences [5]. However, the original DRAMMS defines similarity by the Sum of Squared Differences (SSD) of attributes which limits its application in MR-US multi-modal registration. We propose the Correlation Coefficient (CC) of attributes to better adapt to MR-US multi-modal registration.

2.1 Problem Formulation

In the original DRAMMS formulation, given two images $I_1 : \Omega_1 \mapsto \mathbb{R}$ and $I_2 : \Omega_2 \mapsto \mathbb{R}$ in 3D image domains Ω_i $(i = 1, 2) \subset \mathbb{R}^3$, we seek a transformation T that maps every voxel $\boldsymbol{u} \in \Omega_1$ to its correspondence $\mathrm{T}(\boldsymbol{u}) \in \Omega_2$, by minimizing an overall cost function $E(T)$,

$$\min_T E(T) = \int_{\boldsymbol{u} \in \Omega_1} \underbrace{ms(\boldsymbol{u}, T(\boldsymbol{u}))}_{\text{Mutual-Saliency}} \cdot \underbrace{sim\left(A_1^\star(\boldsymbol{u}), A_2^\star(T(\boldsymbol{u}))\right) d\boldsymbol{u}}_{\text{Attribute Matching}} + \lambda R(T) \qquad (1)$$

where $A_i^\star(\boldsymbol{u})(i = 1, 2)$ is the optimal attribute vector that reflects the geometric and anatomical contexts around voxel $\boldsymbol{u}$, and d is its dimension. The term $ms(\boldsymbol{u}, T(\boldsymbol{u}))$ is a continuously-valued mutual-saliency weight between two voxels $\boldsymbol{u} \in \Omega_1$ and $\mathrm{T}(\boldsymbol{u}) \in \Omega_2$. This way, registration is driving by reliably matched voxel pairs which are not

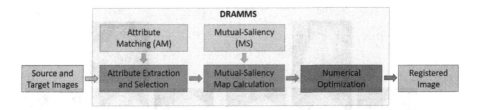

Fig. 1. Non-rigid deformation framework.

necessarily less deformed voxels. The term $R(T)$ is a smoothness/regularization term usually corresponding to the Laplacian operator, or the bending energy, of the deformation field T, whereas λ is a parameter that controls the extent of smoothness. The proposed framework is sketched in Fig. 1.

2.2 Attribute Matching

The aim of attribute matching is to extract and select optimal attributes that reflect the geometric and anatomic contexts of each voxel. It consists of two parts: attribute extraction and attribute selection.

Attribute Extraction. A set of multi-scale and multi-orientation Gabor attributes is extracted at each voxel by convolving the images with a set of Gabor filter banks. The parameter settings developed by [6] were adopted: the number of scales, M, is set to 4 and the number of orientations, N, is set to 6, the highest frequency is set at 0.4 Hz and the lowest frequency at 0.05 Hz. Figure 2 shows an example of multi-scale and multi-orientation Gabor attributes extracted from (a) intraoperative US and (b) preoperative MR images. After attribute extraction, each voxel $\mathbf{u} = (x, y, z)$ is characterized by a Gabor attribute vector $\tilde{A}_1(u)$ with dimension $D = M \times N \times 4$.

Attribute Selection. The aim is to select components of attributes to increase the reliability of matching between two images. An expectation-maximization (EM) framework is used. Given the full-length attributes, the E-step finds spatially-scattered (and hence spatially representative) voxel pairs with not just high similarity but more importantly, reliably high similarity. Then on the selected voxel pairs, M-step uses the iterative forward inclusion and backward elimination (iFIBE) feature selection algorithm to find a subset of attribute components that maximize the similarity and matching reliability (defined as mutual-saliency). A major difference from [4] is that the similarity $sim(\boldsymbol{p}, \boldsymbol{q})$ between a pair of voxels $(\boldsymbol{p} \in \Omega_1, \boldsymbol{q} \in \Omega_2)$ is defined based on the correlation coefficient of their attribute vectors:

$$sim\big(\tilde{A}_1(\boldsymbol{p}), \tilde{A}_2(\boldsymbol{q})\big) = CC\big(\tilde{A}_1(\boldsymbol{p}), \tilde{A}_2(\boldsymbol{q})\big) \in [0, 1] \tag{2}$$

where higher correlation coefficient between to attribute vectors indicates higher similarity.

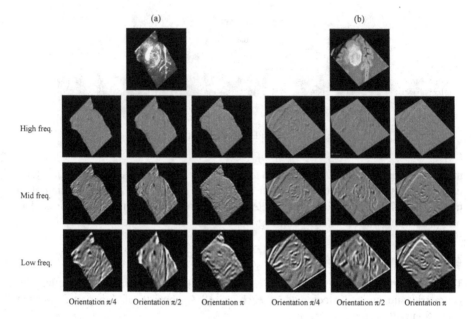

Fig. 2. Multi-scale and multi-orientation Gabor attributes extracted from (a) intraoperative US image and (b) preoperative MR images.

2.3   Mutual-Saliency Map to Modulate Registration

We assign a continuously-valued weight to each voxel, based on the capability of each voxel to establish reliable correspondences across images. This idea is formulated in Eq. (3) and in the associated Fig. 3. Mutual-saliency value, $ms(u, T(u))$, is calculated by dividing the mean similarity between u and all voxels in the core neighborhood (CN) of $T(u)$, with the mean similarity between u and all voxels in the peripheral neighborhood (PN) of $T(u)$.

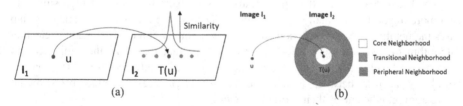

Fig. 3. The idea of mutual-saliency measure: (a) The matching between a pair of voxels **u** and T(**u**) is unique if they are similar to each other and not to anything else in the neighborhood. A delta function in the similarity map indicates a unique matching, and hence high mutual-saliency value. (b) Mutual-saliency function measures the uniqueness of the matching between a voxel pair in a neighborhood. Different colors represent different layers of neighborhoods.

$$ms(\boldsymbol{u}, T(\boldsymbol{u})) = \frac{MEAN_{v \in CN(T(\boldsymbol{u}))}[sim(A_1(\boldsymbol{u}), A_2(\boldsymbol{v}))]}{MEAN_{v \in PN(T(\boldsymbol{u}))}[sim(A_1(\boldsymbol{u}), A_2(\boldsymbol{v}))]} \qquad (3)$$

where sim ($\cdot$, $\cdot$) is the attribute-based similarity between two voxels (Eq. 2). The radius of each neighborhood is adaptive to the scale in which Gabor attributes are extracted. For a typical isotropic 3D brain image, the radius of core, transitional and peripheral neighborhood are 2, 5, 8 voxels, respectively [4].

2.4   Deformation Model and Optimization Strategy

The diffeomorphic FFD [7, 8] is chosen because of its flexibility to handle a smooth and diffeomorphic deformation field. We have chosen discrete optimization, a state-of-the-art optimization strategy known for computational efficiency and robustness regarding local optima [9, 10].

3   Results

Preoperative T2-FLAIR MR and intraoperative predurotomy US images were acquired from 22 patients with low-grade gliomas. A set of 15 to 16 homologous landmarks were identified across images (pre-operative MRI vs. US before resection) and used to

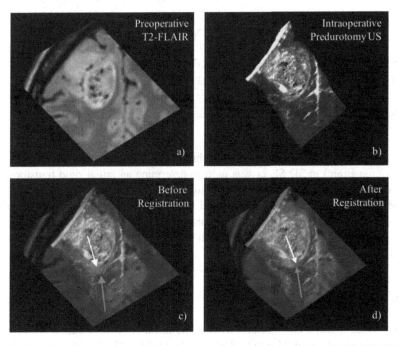

Fig. 4. Preoperative MR to intraoperative US registration. (a) preoperative T2-FLAIR MR and (b) intraoperative US images. Superimposed preoperative MR to intraoperative US (c) before registration and (d) after non-linear correction. Arrows indicate (c) the misalignment between the tumor boundaries in the different modalities and (d) the alignment after registration.

Table 1. Details of inter-modality landmarks for each clinical case. The number of landmarks and the mean initial Euclidean distances between landmark pairs are shown, and the range (min–max) of the distances is shown in parenthesis after the mean value. The last column shows the results after registration.

Case	Number of landmarks	Before registration (mm)	After registration (mm)
1	15	1.82 (0.56–3.84)	1.58 (0.53–3.07)
2	15	5.68 (3.43–8.99)	3.89 (2.05–4.33)
3	15	9.58 (8.57–10.34)	4.92 (1.37–5.01)
4	15	2.99 (1.61–4.55)	2.36 (1.55–3.48)
5	15	12.02 (10.08–14.18)	4.02 (1.92–5.45)
6	15	3.27 (2.27–4.26)	1.51 (0.96–3.21)
7	15	1.82 (0.22–3.63)	1.48 (0.20–3.57)
8	15	2.63 (1.00–4.15)	2.03 (0.83–3.94)
12	16	19.68 (18.53–21.30)	5.59 (1.24–6.47)
13	15	4.57 (2.73–7.52)	3.94 (1.29–4.83)
14	15	3.03 (1.99–4.43)	2.98 (1.99–4.06)
15	15	3.21 (1.15–5.90)	2.65(1.37–5.85)
16	15	3.39 (1.68–4.47)	3.28 (1.68–4.37)
17	16	6.39 (4.46–7.83)	4.78 (3.90–6.05)
18	16	3.56 (1.44–5.47)	3.25 (1.41–4.73)
19	15	3.28 (1.30–5.42)	3.07 (1.22–4.80)
21	15	4.55 (3.44–6.17)	4.51 (2.93–5.29)
23	15	7.01 (5.26–8.26)	4.67 (3.10–5.82)
24	16	1.10 (0.45–2.04)	1.10 (0.37–2.09)
25	15	10.06 (7.10–15.12)	5.55 (2.98–7.04)
26	16	2.83 (1.60–4.40)	1.93 (1.04–3.37)
27	16	5.76 (4.84–7.14)	4.58 (0.98–6.12)
Mean ± Std		5.37 ± 4.27	3.35 ± 1.39

validate the deformable registration algorithm [11]. The Transforms Module (General Registration Brain) in 3D Slicer was used to determine an initial rigid transformation between each pair of images before applying our method. Figure 4 shows an example of one pair of preoperative T2-FLAIR and intraoperative US images and their alignment before and after deformable registration. Table 1 presents the mean target registration error (mTRE) in mm and for each clinical case, before and after deformable registration.

4 Conclusions

The proposed registration algorithm reduces the mean target registration error from an initial value of 5.37 ± 4.27 mm to 3.35 ± 1.19 mm for 22 clinical cases. Our future work includes: (i) further comparison of different similarity measures in MR-US registration, (ii) exploring different linear registration methods to initialize deformable registration, (iii) using blurring and gradient information to reduce the negative influence of speckles in the ultrasound image and (iv) investigating the potential to combine landmark-based to voxel-wise registration.

References

1. Roberts, D., Hartov, A., Kennedy, F., Miga, M., Paulsen, K.: Intraoperative brain shift and deformation: a quantitative analysis of cortical displacement in 28 cases. Neurosurgery **43**, 749–758 (1998)
2. Letteboer, M.M.J., Willems, P.W., Viergever, M.A., Niessen, W.J.: Brain shift estimation in image-guided neurosurgery using 3-D ultrasound. IEEE Trans. Biomed. Eng. **52**(2), 268–276 (2005)
3. Audette, M.A., Siddiqi, K., Ferrie, F.P., Peters, T.M.: An integrated range-sensing, segmentation and registration framework for the characterization of intra-surgical brain deformations in image-guided surgery. Comput. Vis. Image Underst. **89**(2–3), 226–251 (2003)
4. Ou, Y., Sotiras, A., Paragios, N., Davatzikos, C.: DRAMMS: deformable registration via attribute matching and mutual-saliency weighting. Med. Image Anal. **15**(4), 622–639 (2011)
5. Ou, Y., Akbari, H., Bilello, M., Da, X., Davatzikos, C.: Comparative evaluation of registration algorithms in different brain databases with varying difficulty: results and insights. IEEE Trans. Med. Imaging **33**(10), 2039–2065 (2014)
6. Zhan, Y., Shen, D.: Deformable segmentation of 3D ultrasound prostate images using statistical texture matching method. IEEE Trans. Med. Imaging **25**, 256–272 (2006)
7. Rueckert, D., Sonoda, L.I., Hayes, C., Hill, D.L., Leach, M.O., Hawkes, D.J.: Nonrigid registration using free-form deformations: application to breast MR images. IEEE Trans. Med. Imaging **18**(8), 712–721 (1999)
8. Rueckert, D., Aljabar, P., Heckemann, R.A., Hajnal, J.V., Hammers, A.: Diffeomorphic registration using B-splines. In: Larsen, R., Nielsen, M., Sporring, J. (eds.) MICCAI 2006. LNCS, vol. 4191, pp. 702–709. Springer, Heidelberg (2006). https://doi.org/10.1007/11866763_86
9. Komodakis, N., Tziritas, G., Paragios, N.: Performance vs computational efficiency for optimizing single and dynamic MRFs: setting the state of the art with primal-dual strategies. Comput. Vis. Image Underst. **112**(1), 14–29 (2008)
10. Glocker, B., Komodakis, N., Tziritas, G., Navab, N., Paragios, N.: Dense image registration through MRFs and efficient linear programming. Med. Image Anal. **12**(6), 731–741 (2008)
11. Xiao, Y., Fortin, M., Unsgård, G., Rivaz, H., Reinertsen, I.: REtroSpective Evaluation of Cerebral Tumors (RESECT): a clinical database of pre-operative MRI and intra-operative ultrasound in low-grade glioma surgeries. Med. Phys. **44**(7), 3875–3882 (2017)

Registration of MRI and iUS Data to Compensate Brain Shift Using a Symmetric Block-Matching Based Approach

David Drobny[1,2]([⊠]) [iD], Tom Vercauteren[2] [iD], Sébastien Ourselin[2] [iD], and Marc Modat[2] [iD]

[1] Wellcome/EPSRC Centre for Interventional and Surgical Sciences, University College London, London, UK
d.drobny.17@ucl.ac.uk
[2] School of Biomedical Engineering and Imaging Sciences, King's College London, King's Health Partners, St Thomas' Hospital, London SE1 7EH, UK
{tom.vercauteren,sebastien.ourselin,marc.modat}@kcl.ac.uk

Abstract. This paper describes the application of an established block-matching based registration approach to the CuRIOUS 2018 MICCAI registration challenge. Different variations of this method are compared to demonstrate possible results of a fully automatic and general approach. The results can be used as a reference, for example when evaluating the performance of methods that are specifically developed for ultrasound to MRI registration.

Keywords: Brain shift · Fully automatic · MRI · iUS
Symmetric registration · Block-matching

1 Introduction

Update of pre-surgical images and surgery plans to improve the accuracy of displayed information is an active field of research. Intra-operative ultrasound (iUS) is an accessible imaging technique that can be used to acquire data of the brain during a surgery. With these intra-operative images, the brain shift can be estimated via image registration. For the CuRIOUS 2018 MICCAI challenge, we suggest a method which uses a symmetric block-matching approach to fully automatically align the pre-operative MRI with the iUS image. This is an established method whose benefits were shown in different applications [2,3]. The results can then be compared to more specialized approaches in this field.

2 Methods

It has been shown that asymmetric registration algorithms can impair the evaluation of biomarkers, e.g. brain atrophy [9] and should thus be used with caution.

© Springer Nature Switzerland AG 2018
D. Stoyanov et al. (Eds.): POCUS 2018/BIVPCS 2018/CuRIOUS 2018/CPM 2018,
LNCS 11042, pp. 172–178, 2018.
https://doi.org/10.1007/978-3-030-01045-4_21

Direct comparison of an asymmetric and symmetric block-matching framework showed further advantages like improved capture range, higher accuracy and robustness of the symmetric approach [5]. The symmetric registration algorithm used in this comparison is published as part of the NiftyReg open source software package (version 1.5.58) [6] and is applied on this registration challenge (Fig. 1).

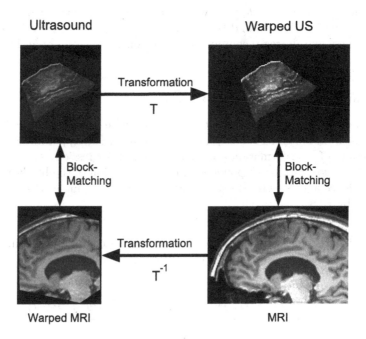

Fig. 1. Overview of the symmetric registration approach. In every registration step the iUS image is warped into the MRI space and vice versa. Block-matching is then performed in the respective domain to update the transformation with the established correspondences. The transformations are averaged to ensure inverse consistency.

2.1   Block-Matching Based Global Registration

The block-Matching method for registration iteratively establishes point correspondences between reference image and the warped floating image and then determines the transformation parameters by least trimmed squares (LTS) regression [7]. The LTS regression only considers 50% of inlier values.

For the block-matching, both images are divided into uniform blocks of 4 voxel edge length. The 25% of blocks with the highest variance of intensity values are used and the rest is discarded. Each of these reference image blocks is compared to all floating image blocks that overlap with at least one voxel (this results in a search space with 7 voxel edge length). The matching block for each reference block is determined as the one with maximum absolute normalized cross correlation (NCC) according to

$$\text{NCC} = \frac{1}{N} \sum_{x \in b_r} \frac{[b_r(x) - \mu_{b_r}] \, [b_f(x) - \mu_{b_f}]}{\sigma_{b_r} \, \sigma_{b_f}}, \tag{1}$$

with the blocks in reference (b_f) and warped image (b_r), the mean μ and standard deviation σ within a block, and the number of voxel in a block N. To increase the robustness and decrease computation time, only a fraction of all blocks are matched.

2.2 Symmetric Registration Extension

The block matching step provides two sets of point-wise correspondences between the images: from image I to J $\{C_{I \to J}\}$ and vice versa $\{C_{J \to I}\}$. The second step is the update of transformation parameters via LTS regression. At every iteration $i+1$ and for both correspondences, the composition of the block-matching correspondence and the previous transformation $T^{(i)}$ determines the new transformation by LTS:

$$T^{(i+1)} = \text{LTS}[C \circ T^{(i)}]. \tag{2}$$

To ensure inverse consistency (i.e. $T_{I \to J} \equiv T_{J \to I}^{-1}$) at each update, the directional transformation matrices of the LTS regression are averaged according to [1]:

$$T_{I \to J}^{(i+1)} = \text{expm} \left(\frac{\text{logm} \left(\text{LTS} \left[T_{I \to J}^{(i)} \circ C_{I \to J} \right] \right) + \text{logm} \left(\text{LTS} \left[T_{J \to I}^{(i)} \circ C_{J \to I} \right]^{-1} \right)}{2} \right) \tag{3}$$

$$T_{J \to I}^{(i+1)} = \text{expm} \left(\frac{\text{logm} \left(\text{LTS} \left[T_{J \to I}^{(i)} \circ C_{J \to I} \right] \right) + \text{logm} \left(\text{LTS} \left[T_{I \to J}^{(i)} \circ C_{I \to J} \right]^{-1} \right)}{2} \right), \tag{4}$$

where expm and logm are the exponential and logarithmic matrix operators, respectively.

2.3 Experiments

The NiftyReg software is based on the NIfTI-1.1 file format so that the MINC files of the RESECT database [8] have to be converted first. We used the MINC tools provided by the McConnell Brain Imaging Centre, Montreal Neurological Institute at McGill University [4] for the conversion. The initial alignment of iUS and MRI images (based on tracking of the iUS probe) are derived from the header information. This alignment is the baseline and the corresponding results are referenced to as initial. Masks derived from thresholding the iUS image at an intensity value of 0 (i.e. masking out the background) and dilating the result by 10 voxels are used for all registrations. Then the described block-matching based registration is applied with a 2 level pyramidal approach. On the first level, 10 iterations are computed, on the finer level only 5. The symmetric approach is evaluated once with the T1-weighted MRI (symm-T1) and once with the FLAIR MRI (symm-FLAIR). These approaches are compared to the four asymmetric approaches: with the iUS image as reference and the T1-MRI as floating image (asymm-US-T1) and vice-versa (asymm-T1-US) as well as with the iUS image as reference and the FLAIR-MRI as floating image (asymm-US-FLAIR) and vice-versa (asymm-FLAIR-US). These 6 approaches are each computed with a rigid and affine transformation. Furthermore the affine transformation that minimizes the target registration error (TRE) is included in the comparison as an optimal result (affine oracle).

3   Results

For all described approaches, the average of all case specific mean TREs is computed as an overall measure of registration accuracy. The results are summarized in Table 1. It can be seen that the symmetric approach using the FLAIR data, symm-FLAIR, as well as the asymmetric approach asymm-T1-US fail and increase the TRE. The best approaches are asymm-US-FLAIR, asymm-US-T1 and symm-T1. The asymm-US-FLAIR approach shows the best results reducing the initial average TRE of 5.37 mm to 3.77 mm and 2.90 mm with rigid and affine registration respectively, improving 20 and 18 out of the 22 cases. For asymm-US-T1 the TRE is reduced to 4.34 mm and 3.78 mm, improving 15 and 17 out of the 22 cases with rigid and affine registration, respectively. The symm-T1 approach shows good results with an average TRE of 3.84 mm, on par with the asymm-US-T1 affine. This symmetric approach improved the TRE for 18 of 22 cases.

Table 1. Average mean TRE in mm and 95% confidence interval for all tested approaches.

	Initial	Rigid	Affine	Affine oracle
asymm-US-T1	5.37 [3.48, 7.27]	4.34 [2.71, 5.96]	3.78 [2.36, 5.19]	0.95 [0.88, 1.02]
asymm-T1-US		8.49 [6.41, 10.57]	16.15 [10.95, 21.36]	
symm-T1		3.84 [2.10, 5.57]	5.41 [4.48, 6.34]	
asymm-US-FLAIR		3.77 [1.91, 5.64]	2.90 [1.31, 4.49]	
asymm-FLAIR-US		8.84 [6.49, 11.18]	16.52 [11.52, 21.52]	
symm-FLAIR		8.75 [6.48, 11.02]	13.50 [9.05, 17.96]	

In a few cases, the initial alignment has rather large TREs which are not fully recovered by the approaches although the optimal computed transformation shows that an affine transformation is able to reduce the TRE to values similar to

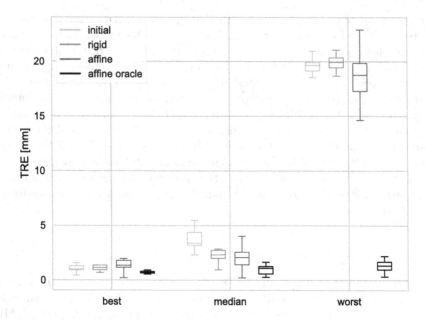

Fig. 2. Boxplots showing TRE results for best-, median- and worst-case subjects of initial, asymm-US-FLAIR rigid, asymm-US-FLAIR affine, and affine oracle (from left to right within each group).

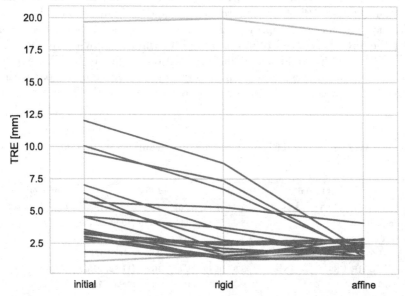

Fig. 3. Spaghetti-plot showing the mean TRE for every case with the initial position and the asymm-US-FLAIR approach with both rigid and affine registration. Blue lines indicate an decrease of the mean TRE by the rigid registration approach, red lines an increase. (Color figure online)

the other cases. Figure 2 visualizes the TRE distribution for 4 approaches (init, symm-T1 rig, symm-T1 aff, and opt) with 3 cases each: the best, the median and the worst case (determined by average mean TRE). Comparing the affine and the rigid approach, the affine increases the TRE on average and especially for cases with lower initial TRE. On the other hand, the TRE of the worst cases is reduced most by the affine approach. This can be seen in Fig. 3 where each line represents the mean TRE of an individual case. Most lines decrease from initial value to the rigid result before increasing to the affine result while the three cases with initial highest TRE decrease with the affine approach.

4   Discussion

We have demonstrated that a fully automated standard registration approach can reduce the average mean TRE of the given data set from 5.37 mm to 2.90 mm (using the asymmetric approach with the iUS image as reference and the FLAIR MRI image as floating image). One other asymmetric approach and a symmetric approach achieved acceptable results while the other considered approaches could not improve the registration accuracy. The given data set includes one outlier case with a very high initial TRE, which is not improved much in most approaches. Excluding this case yields even better results with 2.15 mm average mean TRE for asymm-US-FLAIR affine. These results require no user interaction and rely mostly on default parameters. Comparing the results to an optimal transformation based on matching the given landmark correspondences, it becomes clear that results could be improved further. Changes of, for example the similarity measure or pre-processing steps could be adapted for this registration problem. Furthermore the combination of the information of both MRI images into a multi-spectral registration approach could improve the results.

Acknowledgments. D. Drobny is supported by the UCL EPSRC Centre for Doctoral Training in Medical Imaging and Wellcome/EPSRC Centre for Interventional and Surgical Sciences [NS/A000050/1]. This work is also supported by the Wellcome/EPSRC Centre for Medical Engineering [WT 203148/Z/16/Z] and EPSRC [NS/A000027/1].

References

1. Alexa, M.: Linear combination of transformations. ACM Trans. Graph. **21**(3) (2002). https://doi.org/10.1145/566654.566592
2. Ebner, M., et al.: Volumetric reconstruction from printed films: enabling 30 year longitudinal analysis in MR neuroimaging. NeuroImage **165**, 238–250 (2018)
3. Markiewicz, P.J., et al.: NiftyPET: a high-throughput software platform for high quantitative accuracy and precision PET imaging and analysis. Neuroinformatics **16**(1), 95–115 (2017)
4. mnc2nii GitHub page. https://github.com/BIC-MNI/minc-tools/blob/master/conversion/nifti1/mnc2nii.c. Accessed 29 June 2018
5. Modat, M., Cash, D.M., Daga, P., Winston, G.P., Duncan, J.S., Ourselin, S.: Global image registration using a symmetric block-matching approach. J. Med. Imaging (Bellingham) **1**(2), 024003 (2014)

6. NiftyReg GitHub page. https://github.com/KCL-BMEIS/niftyreg/wiki. Accessed 29 June 2018
7. Ourselin, S., Roche, A., Subsol, G., Pennec, X., Ayache, N.: Reconstructing a 3D structure from serial histological sections. Image Vis. Comput. **19**(1–2), 25–31 (2001). https://doi.org/10.1016/s0262-8856(00)00052-4
8. Yiming, X., Maryse, F., Geirmund, U., Hassan, R., Ingerid, R.: REtroSpective Evaluation of Cerebral Tumors (RESECT): a clinical database of pre-operative MRI and intra-operative ultrasound in low-grade glioma surgeries. Med. Phys. **44**(7), 3875–3882 (2017)
9. Yushkevich, P.A., Avants, B.B., Das, S.R., Pluta, J., Altinay, M., Craige, C.: Bias in estimation of hippocampal atrophy using deformation-based morphometry arises from asymmetric global normalization: an illustration in ADNI 3T MRI data. NeuroImage **50**(2), 434–445 (2010)

Intra-operative Brain Shift Correction with Weighted Locally Linear Correlations of 3DUS and MRI

Roozbeh Shams[1], Marc-Antoine Boucher[1], and Samuel Kadoury[1,2(✉)]

[1] MedICAL Laboratory, Polytechnique Montreal, Montreal, Canada
samuel.kadoury@polymtl.ca
[2] CHUM Research Center, Montreal, QC, Canada

Abstract. During brain tumor resection procedures, 3D ultrasound (US) can be used to assess brain shift, as intra-operative MRI is challenging due to immobilization issues, and may require sedation. Brain shift can cause uncertainty in the localization of resected tumor margins and deviate the registered pre-operative MRI surgical plan. Hence, 3D US can be used to compensate for the deformation. The objective of this study is to propose an approach to automatically register the patient's MRI to intra-operative 3D US using a deformable registration approach based on a weighted adaptation of the locally linear correlation metric for US-MRI fusion, adapting both hyper-echoic and hypo-echoic regions within the cortex. Evaluation was performed on a cohort of 23 patients, where 3D US and MRI were acquired on the same day. The proposed approach demonstrates a statistically significant improvement of internal landmark localization made by expert radiologists, with a mean target registration error (mTRE) of 4.6 ± 3.4 mm, compared to an initial mTRE of 5.3 ± 4.2 mm, demonstrating the clinical benefit of this tool to correct for brain shift using 3D ultrasound.

1 Introduction

One of the key challenges facing brain resection surgeries and accurate localisation of the structure of interest during epilepsy surgery is the estimation of the soft tissue deformation (known as brain shift) that can occur due to brain swelling, craniotomy, tumor mass effects or surgical resection. Brain shift can lead to nonlinear deformation of the anatomy and cause the planned structures of interest to significantly shift during surgery, either directly over or around the tumor. In order to predict soft organ deformation, recent studies have resorted to multichannel anatomical and fractional anisotropy algorithms [1] as well as to non-linear finite element modelling [2]. These studies have however only been tested on adult populations and heavily rely on using interventional MRI to survey this effect during surgery. The use of commercially available stereotactic optical tracking systems also has limitations with respect to surface-based registration [3] and precise tip localization of the subdural electrodes inside the brain

© Springer Nature Switzerland AG 2018
D. Stoyanov et al. (Eds.): POCUS 2018/BIVPCS 2018/CuRIOUS 2018/CPM 2018,
LNCS 11042, pp. 179–184, 2018.
https://doi.org/10.1007/978-3-030-01045-4_22

tissue with visually assessing the penetration near the sylvian fissure. Ultra-sonography may circumvent these limitations by implementing methods which allow metallic tool tip tracking using sensor responses [4] and inferring shape morphology based on transcranial US imaging of soft tissue for registration pur-poses. Hence, the problems of reliable fiducialess image-based registration, non-rigid brain shift due to craniotomy or resection, and accurate tool tracking in deep sub-cortical structures during neurosurgery in children remain unsolved, and could potentially be alleviated with ultrasonography.

The use of high-order structural priors have also been attempted to maintain anatomical warping coherency due to the presence of multiple local minima. These methods were applied in scenarios using baseline registration near the occipital lobe where standard stereotactic methods fail due to lacking salient topological features on the cranial surface, and to potential brain shift com-pensation caused by tumor resection, craniotomy or fluid drainage in patients undergoing surgery by using texture features for automatic alignment [5].

In this paper, we present a novel method to correct for intra-operative brain shift from 3D US images. Multi-modal images of the same patient are automati-cally registered from patient's MRI to intra-operative 3D US using a deformable registration approach based on a weighted adaptation of the locally linear corre-lation metric for US-MRI fusion, computing weights for the hypoechoic area and the hyperechoic area. Results are compared with ground truth manual identifica-tion of landmarks on MRI and 3DUS images, demonstrating the clinical potential in neurosurgery to quantify displacement of internal brain tissue. The contribu-tion is the introduction of a novel optimization scheme based on a dynamic weighting factor in the fusion process, handling hyper and hypo-echoic regions within the cortical regions with a multimodal similarity metric [6].

2   Brain Shift Compensation Method

The first step of the brain shift compensation method is an initialization pro-cedure, where the patient's MRI is globally positioned to the patient's 3D US image. This is followed by a rigid and non-rigid registration step, using a locally linear correlation metric with dynamic weighted technique to account for varying level of echogenicity in the cortex.

Initialization. The orientation of the US images is first corrected by rotat-ing the volume to match the orientation observed on the MRI volume. This is performed from a PCA on the extracted inferior skull region, to identify the principal orientation vectors of the head. Then, the brain in 3D US is extracted with the method and its center position and size are calculated. Based on those measurements, a scaling and a translation are applied to the MRI atlases before the registration.

Multimodal MRI/3D US Registration. Multimodal registration between 3DUS and MRI images is performed with a locally linear correlation metric

(LC^2) by [6] which correlates MRI intensities and gradients with US intensities. This fusion step is achieved in a patch-based approach of US voxels compared to intensity and gradient magnitude information extracted from the MRI using the relationship:

$$f(x_i) = \alpha p_i + \beta g_i + \gamma \tag{1}$$

with x_i as the voxel intensity in $\mathcal{I}_{3DUS}$, T_{def} the deformation field, $p_i = p(T_{def}(x_i))$ and $g_i = |\nabla p_i|$ are the intensity and gradient magnitude at the corresponding voxel in the moving image. We define the values $c = \{\alpha, \beta, \gamma\}$ for all voxels x_i determined with a 3D region Ω_i of m voxels. This cubic region of size $7 \times 7 \times 7$ ($m = 343$) surrounding x_i is used to minimize $(f(x_i) - \mathcal{I}_{3DUS}(x_i))$ on Ω_i with a LMS minimization process of c as shown below:

$$c = (M^T M)^{-1} M^T U \tag{2}$$

$$\text{where } M = \begin{pmatrix} p_1 & g_1 & 1 \\ \vdots & \vdots & \vdots \\ p_m & g_m & 1 \end{pmatrix}, U = \begin{pmatrix} \mathcal{I}_{3DUS}(x_1) \\ \vdots \\ \mathcal{I}_{3DUS}(x_m) \end{pmatrix} \tag{3}$$

with $\mathcal{I}_{3DUS}(x_{\{1,...,m\}})$ as the US voxels in Ω_i, with $p_{\{1,...,m\}}$ and $g_{\{1,...,m\}}$ the intensities and gradients of the corresponding MR voxels. The closeness measurement obtained locally is then estimated on Ω_i with:

$$\Theta_i^2(u, f) = 1 - \frac{\sum_{\Omega_i} |\mathcal{I}_{3DUS}(x_i) - f(x_i)|^2}{m \cdot Var(\mathcal{I}_{3DUS}(x_i)|x_i \in \Omega_i)} \tag{4}$$

where $f(x_i)$ is as defined in Eq.(1) with $c = \{\alpha, \beta, \gamma\}$, previously determined for Ω_i by Eq. (2). Here, $Var(\mathcal{I}_{3DUS}(x_i)|x_i \in \Omega_i)$ is the variance of the US intensities over Ω_i.

The general measurement Θ^2 includes a pondered summation in Eq. (4) of all points x_i, using as weights the standard-deviation of US voxel intensities. Furthermore, to simplify the computational complexity and focus only on relevant voxels belonging to the cortical areas in the MRI and US, we constrain the matching of voxel within a pre-segmented mask of the brain region, which excludes any background intensities from the similarity measure. Consequently, only the US intensities x_i corresponding to moving voxels within the MRI affects the brain shift compensation.

The non-rigid deformation field T_{def} is controlled by a cubic $5 \times 5 \times 5$ B-Spline interpolation grid, distributed in a uniform fashion within the fan-shape region of the $\mathcal{I}_{3DUS}$. The optimization of the registration (i.e. maximization of Θ^2) is performed using a bound optimization by quadratic approximations, as it avoids the analytic form of the Θ^2 derivative, but rather performs an approximation during the minimization process.

The registration includes a rigid step with LC^2 and non-rigid step with $LC^2 + P$ where P is a pixel weighting term. P is a term created specifically to describe brain regions in US by making use of the hypoechoic area (fluid cavities) and the hyperechoic area (ex. choroid plexus). Since only the US voxels included in the MRI label are analyzed, P is only added at the non-rigid registration step when the MRI labels are already roughly aligned to the US image:

$$P = \frac{C_1 \sum_{i=1}^{N} \epsilon_i max(I_L - I(v_i), 0) + (1 - \epsilon_i)max(I(v_i) - I_H, 0) + C_2}{N} \quad (5)$$

where $\epsilon_i = 1$ when v_i is in the hypoechoic area and $\epsilon_i = 0$ when v_i is in the hyperechoic area, C_1, C_2 are coefficients adjusted to the intensities and N is the number of voxels in the MRI volume. Moreover, P is adjusted to penalize smaller labels (which statistically have higher P) $P_{adj}(V_k) = P(\frac{V_k}{V_M})^{\frac{1}{4}}$ where V_k is the active label volume and V_m the mean label volume.

This term is added only at the non-rigid step because it is highly specific to the internal areas in US such as the lateral ventricles which were roughly aligned to the US ventricles. In cerebral ultrasound, the most hypoechoic and the most hyperechoic regions correspond to the lateral ventricles fluid cavities and the choroid plexus, respectively. The two areas are each defined by a threshold and constrained within a region of interest centered at the middle of the brain. Considering the whole volume, the hyperechoic area is constrained to the posterior part representing 60% of the volume and the hypoechoic to the anterior part (60% of the volume) or the superior part (25% of the volume).

Optimization Strategy. The optimization of the registration process was performed using BOBYQA from [7] as proposed in [6], which does not require the metric's derivatives. Registration is repeated $N = 100$ and a selection of the top ranking ($n = 4$) exemplars is performed based on the resulting similarity metric.

3   Results

In this study, a subset of 22 cases out of 23 adult patients with low-grade gliomas (Grade II) were included, with 3D US and T1 weighted MRI acquired for all patients during the same day. Ultrasound images were acquired with a linear probe (6–12 MHz) with a 48×13 mm footprint and reconstructed in 3D using the optically tracked positions of the ultrasound probe, while the MRI was acquired with both 1.5 T and 3T Siemens MR scanners, with 12 and 20 channel head coils respectively, an image resolution of 256×256, and pixel size of $1.0 \times 1.0 \times 1.0$ mm. Markers were used for baseline image-to-patient registration after head immobilization on the operating table. A detailed description of the dataset is provided in [8].

The accuracy was assessed using expert manual landmark identification on US and MRI. The correlation between the ground truth locations and the automatically registered landmarks was $r = 0.921$. The results were compared to registrations accomplished with the original LC^2 metric and the STAPLE [9] method in order to non-rigidly register the MRI to the 3D US reconstructed volume. Table 1 summarizes the results with the mean target registration error (mTRE), before and after brain shift correction. The results demonstrate a statistically significant improvement from the initial registration using the proposed

Table 1. Comparison in accuracy and execution time of the registration methods from 3D US, based on target registration errors (TRE).

Methods	Initial mTRE (mm)	Final mTRE (mm)	Time (sec)
Original LC^2 [6]	5.3 ± 4.2	7.4 ± 5.2	87 ± 11
STAPLE [9]	5.3 ± 4.2	8.7 ± 6.0	434 ± 38
Proposed method	5.3 ± 4.2	**4.6 ± 3.4**	103 ± 12

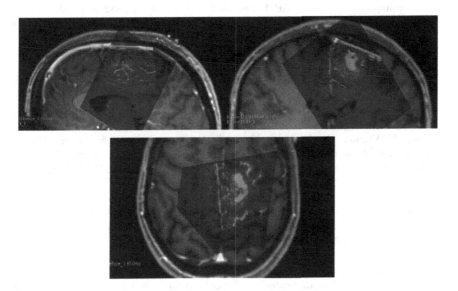

Fig. 1. Sample results of MRI/3DUS registration on case #12.

method based on a paired T-test ($p = 0.005$ for mTRE measures). On the other hand, there were no statistically significant improvement before and after registration using either LC^2 or STAPLE. Figure 1 illustrates an example of the registration results of the MRI and 3DUS.

4 Conclusion

In this paper, we presented an automatic method to perform intra-operative brain shift correction from 3D ultrasound in tumor resection patients. This allows for an automatic correction of registration discrepancies caused by the opening of the dura. Compared to other well established multi-modal registration techniques, the localization of internal landmarks yielded a high correlation with manual identification and indicate statistically significant improvement of the alignment between both modalities. Our main contribution is the introduction of a weighting factor in the modality simulation metric which enables to cope with varying hyper and hypo-echogenicity within the cortex. Future work would include adding a feature learning approach and an extensive validation with additional subjects, both with higher variability in internal deformations, and investigate the use of convolutional neural networks.

References

1. Daga, P., et al.: Accurate localization of optic radiation during neurosurgery in an interventional MRI suite. IEEE Trans. Med. Imaging **31**(4), 882–891 (2012)
2. Wittek, A., Joldes, G., Couton, M., Warfield, S.K., Miller, K.: Patient-specific non-linear finite element modelling for predicting soft organ deformation in real-time; application to non-rigid neuroimage registration. Prog. Biophysics Mol. Biol. **103**(2–3), 292–303 (2010)
3. Mascott, C.R., Sol, J.C., Bousquet, P., Lagarrigue, J., Lazorthes, Y., Lauwers-Cances, V.: Quantification of true in vivo (application) accuracy in cranial image-guided surgery: influence of mode of patient registration. Oper. Neurosurg. **59**(Suppl-1), ONS-146 (2006)
4. Mung, J., Vignon, F., Jain, A.: A non-disruptive technology for robust 3D tool tracking for ultrasound-guided interventions. In: Fichtinger, G., Martel, A., Peters, T. (eds.) MICCAI 2011. LNCS, vol. 6891, pp. 153–160. Springer, Heidelberg (2011). https://doi.org/10.1007/978-3-642-23623-5_20
5. Qiu, W., et al.: Automatic segmentation approach to extracting neonatal cerebral ventricles from 3D ultrasound images. Med. Image Anal. **35**, 181–191 (2017)
6. Fuerst, B., Wein, W., Müller, M., Navab, N.: Automatic ultrasound-MRI registration for neurosurgery using the 2D and 3D LC2 Metric. Med. Image Anal. **18**(8), 1312–1319 (2014)
7. Powell, M.J.: The BOBYQA algorithm for bound constrained optimization without derivatives, pp. 26–46. Cambridge NA Report NA2009/06, University of Cambridge, Cambridge (2009)
8. Xiao, Y., Fortin, M., Unsgård, G., Rivaz, H., Reinertsen, I.: REtroSpective Evaluation of Cerebral Tumors (RESECT): a clinical database of pre-operative MRI and intra-operative ultrasound in low-grade glioma surgeries. Med. Phys. **44**(7), 3875–3882 (2017)
9. Warfield, S.K., Zou, K.H., Wells, W.M.: Simultaneous truth and performance level estimation (STAPLE): an algorithm for the validation of image segmentation. IEEE Trans. Med. Imaging **23**(7), 903–921 (2004)

International Workshop on Computational Precision Medicine, CPM 2018

Survival Modeling of Pancreatic Cancer with Radiology Using Convolutional Neural Networks

Hassan Muhammad[1,2]([⊠]), Ida Häggström[2], David S. Klimstra[2], and Thomas J. Fuchs[1,2]

[1] Weill Cornell Medicine, New York, NY, USA
[2] Memorial Sloan-Kettering Cancer Center, New York, NY, USA
ham2024@med.cornell.edu

Abstract. No reliable biomarkers for early detection of pancreatic cancer are known to date but morphological signatures from non-invasive imaging might be able to close this gap. In this paper, we present a convolutional neural network-based survival model trained directly from computed tomography (CT) images. 159 CT images with associated survival data, and 3D segmentations of organ and tumor were provided by the Pancreatic Cancer Survival Prediction MICCAI grand challenge. A simple, yet novel, approach was used to convert CT slices into RGB-channel images in order to utilize pre-training of the model's convolutional layers. The proposed model achieves a concordance index of 0.85, indicating a relationship between high-level features in CT imaging and disease progression. The ultimate hope is that these promising results translate to more personalized treatment decisions and better cancer care for patients.

Keywords: Deep learning · Radiomics · Survival analysis

1 Introduction

Pancreatic ductal adenocarcinoma (PDAC), commonly referred to as "pancreatic cancer" is the most common neoplasm of the pancreas, affecting approximately 55,000 patients in the US each year. It is also one of the most deadly human cancers and is the 4th leading cause of cancer death in both men and women. The incidence of pancreas cancer has nearly doubled in the last 30 years [10]. Advances in understanding the genomic basis of the disease have not yet translated into more effective treatments, since most patients present with advanced disease, incurable by surgery. However, emerging evidence demonstrates that certain uncommon genomic subtypes are more amenable to targeted chemotherapy, such as those with a BRCA signature or with microsatellite instability [6,8]. A better understanding of the precursor lesions to invasive PDAC also has promise

© Springer Nature Switzerland AG 2018
D. Stoyanov et al. (Eds.): POCUS 2018/BIVPCS 2018/CuRIOUS 2018/CPM 2018,
LNCS 11042, pp. 187–192, 2018.
https://doi.org/10.1007/978-3-030-01045-4_23

to allow advanced diagnostic techniques for early detection [1]. Understanding how the morphology of PDAC reflects the underlying genomic alterations, and how the precursor lesions progress to invasive carcinoma, remain important research objectives. The use of computational analysis to explore subtle morphology clues can provide significant insights into these important issues. Recent advances in deep learning-based survival analysis on histology have paved the way for a robust and direct analysis of medical images in relation to prognosis [9]. Here we offer a similar approach, however for the first time, using 3D radiology to model PDAC prognosis in a novel way.

2   Methods

2.1   Survival Modeling

In most cases, classification or classical regression cannot be used to predict disease prognosis. Survival data suffers what is known as right-censoring where the natural time to event, time to death for example, may be unknown. This can be due to multiple external factors such as a study ending before some deaths have occurred, or a subject dying of a non-disease-related cause. However, time duration until censoring is still useful information which can be included in a survival model. The standard way to model a dataset with right-censored samples is using a Cox proportional hazard model (CPH), as described in Eq. (1) where $\lambda(t|x)$ describes the risk of instantaneous death (hazard) occurring at time t as a function of covariates x, their associated weights β, and a baseline hazard function $\lambda_o(t)$.

$$\lambda(t|x) = \lambda_o(t)\lambda_\beta(x) = \lambda_o(t)exp(\sum_{i=1}^{n} \beta_i x_i) \tag{1}$$

As illustrated by Eq. (2), the CPH regression is performed by tuning β to optimize the Cox partial likelihood which is a product of the probability at each event time T_i that death has occurred to subject i, given the set of subjects $\Re(T_i)$ still at risk. E_i indicates if the event has occurred (censored or not) and the likelihood product is defined over the set of patients with uncensored events $(E_i = 1)$.

$$L(\beta) = \prod_{i:E_i=1} \frac{exp(\beta_i x_i)}{\sum_{j \in \Re(T_i)} exp(\beta_i x_i)} \tag{2}$$

CPH modeling is, however, constrained to linear data and fails when assessing non-linear data such as medical images, which are complex and require a more robust model. In this paper, we construct a survival model which combines a deep convolutional neural network (CNN) and CPH to predict hazard by directly using CT image slice data as covariates. Network weights θ replace β in the CPH model, similar to an approach first described by Farragi [3].

2.2   Network Architecture and Optimization

The CNN architecture used is a replication of AlexNet [7] with some modification. The model is pre-trained on ImageNet data [2] and then has its terminal linear layers customized to predict hazard, similar to CPH. The fully connected layers are replaced with four untrained fully connected layers containing 4096, 1000, 256, and 1 node(s), respectively. This is visualized in Fig. 1. The final node is analogous to $\lambda_\beta(x)$ where weights θ from the 256-layer produce a risk $\lambda_\theta(x)$ to be optimized by the negative log partial likelihood of Eq. (2) as described in Eq. (3).

$$L(\theta) = -\sum(\lambda_\theta(x_i) - log \sum_{j \in \mathcal{R}(T_i)} exp(\lambda_\theta(x_j))) \tag{3}$$

2.3   Experiment

Data dataset used in this study was curated by the MICCAI 2018 Computational Precision Medicine Organizing Committee and was publicly made available through the Pancreatic Cancer Survival Prediction Challenge. The dataset features 159 patients who underwent Pancreas resection at Memorial Sloan Kettering Cancer Center. All patients received contrast enhanced pancreas computed tomography (CT) scans with the organ and tumor manually segmented.

Pre-processing. The CT patient images were all of transaxial size 512×512, with varying number of slices, voxel sizes, and slice thicknesses. All images were thus first resampled to equal voxel size (incl. slice thickness), using nearest interpolation, and then cropped to equal transaxial matrix size of 512×512. Finally, in order to take advantage of the robustness of a pre-trained network, the patient images were again resampled to a transaxial matrix size of 224×224. We generated 224×224 RGB-channel *.png images from the CT data slices to match

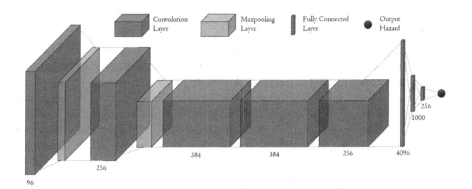

Fig. 1. The model features five convolution layers with maxpooling applied on the first two layers. The output is a single number which functions as an estimation of hazard.

the format of ImageNet, the dataset used for pre-training. The red, blue, and green channels contained a slice of the entire segmented organ, the associated slice of segmented tumor, and a blank matrix of ones respectively. Such an image was generated for each slice of each CT scan, resulting in 4900 images ready for model training. Figure 2 illustrates this process.

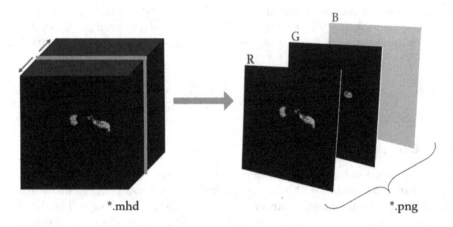

Fig. 2. A 3-channel RGB *.png image is produced from for slice from the CT volume data. The segmented organ is used in the red channel, the segmented tumor in the green channel, and a blank matrix in the blue channel. These RGB images are then used for model training. (Color figure online)

Radiomic Features. Binary tumor masks were created for all images, with value 1 for all nonbackground voxels ($\geq$1000 HU), and 0 for background. Radiomics features were extracted for the tumor data, both for the whole 3D volume, and slice by slice in 2D, using the Pyradiomics package [4]. A total of 70 features were used, based on first order statistics, shape, and textures based on the gray level co-occurrence matrix, and gray level size zone matrix.

Model Training. Each slice in a CT image is treated as an independent training example, and the subject's time to event and event indicator are associated with all slices from the patient's CT image. A training epoch is defined by inputting all converted slices, radiomic features, and survival information from all scans into the model once, each producing a float value representing hazard. While training radiomic image features are concatenated to the first linear layer of the CNN. All hazards for each converted slice in a given scan are averaged to represent a subject's overall hazard. Training epochs are repeated until loss convergence is reached. Stochastic gradient descent with Nesterov momentum is used to minimize $L(\theta)$ with a learning rate of $1e^{-3}$, decreasing one order of magnitude every 20 epochs. In early phases of training, when the hazard output is too large, the $exp(\lambda_\theta(x_j))$ term in the loss function becomes too large, causing an exploding gradient. Using a weight decay of $1e^{-2}$ and gradient clipping helps stabilize the model and allows it to continue training toward convergence.

To assess model performance during training, concordance index (c-index), as described by Harrell [5], is measured at every epoch. The c-index is a commonly used metric to measure survival model's performance in ordering time to death. A c-index of 0.5 indicates a random model while a c-index approaching 1.0 describes a perfect model.

3 Results and Discussion

Figure 3 (top) shows loss decreasing as the model is trained over 50 epochs. This convergence indicates that the model is learning appropriately. In the same

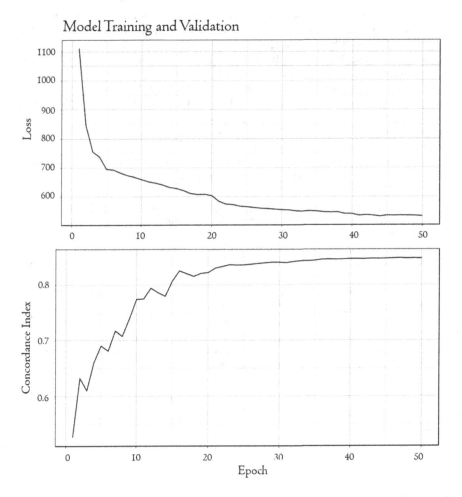

Fig. 3. (Top) loss decreases over training epochs and converges at epoch 50. (Bottom) C-Index increases over training epochs and tapers at 0.85

figure (bottom) c-index can be seen increasing and converging to 0.85 as loss decreases, showing the model improving over epochs. Performance tapers at around 50 epochs.

4   Conclusion

This study shows that a deep CNN survival model can be trained directly on CT image data and perform well. Further work is needed to understand which regions of the CT image correlate most strongly with survival.

References

1. Basturk, O., et al.: A revised classification system and recommendations from the baltimore consensus meeting for neoplastic precursor lesions in the pancreas. Am. J. Surg. Pathol. **39**(12), 1730 (2015)
2. Deng, J., Dong, W., Socher, R., Li, L.J., Li, K., Fei-Fei, L.: ImageNet: a large-scale hierarchical image database. In: IEEE Conference on Computer Vision and Pattern Recognition, 2009, CVPR 2009, pp. 248–255. IEEE (2009)
3. Faraggi, D., Simon, R.: A neural network model for survival data. Stat. Med. **14**(1), 73–82 (1995)
4. van Griethuysen, J.J., et al.: Computational radiomics system to decode the radiographic phenotype. Cancer Res. **77**(21), e104–e107 (2017)
5. Harrell Jr., F.E., Lee, K.L., Califf, R.M., Pryor, D.B., Rosati, R.A.: Regression modelling strategies for improved prognostic prediction. Stat. Med. **3**(2), 143–152 (1984)
6. Kieler, M., Unseld, M., Bianconi, D., Prager, G.: Challenges and perspectives for immunotherapy in adenocarcinoma of the pancreas: the cancer immunity cycle. Pancreas **47**(2), 142–157 (2018)
7. Krizhevsky, A., Sutskever, I., Hinton, G.E.: ImageNet classification with deep convolutional neural networks. In: Advances in Neural Information Processing Systems, pp. 1097–1105 (2012)
8. Lowery, M.A., et al.: Phase II trial of veliparib in patients with previously treated BRCA-mutated pancreas ductal adenocarcinoma. Eur. J. Cancer **89**, 19–26 (2018)
9. Mobadersany, P., et al.: Predicting cancer outcomes from histology and genomics using convolutional networks. Proc. Natl. Acad. Sci., 201717139 (2018)
10. Wu, W., et al.: Rising trends in pancreatic cancer incidence and mortality in 2000–2014. Clin. Epidemiol. **10**, 789–797 (2018)

Pancreatic Cancer Survival Prediction Using CT Scans and Clinical Variables

Li Sun[✉] and Songtao Zhang

Southern University of Science and Technology, Shenzhen 518055, China
`lisun97@foxmail.com`

Abstract. Pancreatic cancer resulted in 411,600 deaths globally in 2015. Pancreatic ductal adenocarcinoma (PDAC) is the most common type of pancreatic cancer and it is highly lethal. Survival for patients with PDAC is dismal due to its aggressive nature, thus the development of novel and reliable prognostic model for early detection and therapy is much desired. Here we proposed a prognostic framework for prediction of overall survival of PDAC patients based on predictors derived from pancreas CT scans and patient clinical variables. Our framework includes three parts: feature extraction, feature selection and survival prediction. First, 2436 radiomics features were extracted from CT scans and were combined with the clinical variables, and a Cox model was fitted to each covariate individually to select the most predictive features. The optimal cut-off was determined by cross-validation. Finally, gradient boosting with component-wise Cox's proportional hazards model was utilized to predict the overall survival of patients. Our framework achieves excellent performance on MICCAI 2018 Pancreatic Cancer Survival Prediction Challenge dataset, achieving mean concordance index of 0.7016 using five-fold cross-validation.

Keywords: Pancreatic cancer · Survival analysis · Prognostic model

1 Introduction

It is estimated that in the United States there are more than 50,000 new cases of pancreatic cancer occur each year, which accounts for about 3% of all cancers in the US and about 7% of all cancer deaths [6]. Pancreatic ductal adenocarcinoma (PDAC) is the most common type of pancreatic cancer, making up more than 80% of cases. It originates in cells lining small tubes in the pancreas called ducts, which transport juices containing important digestive enzymes into the small intestine [1]. Despite substantial research efforts and gradual diagnostic and therapeutic improvements, pancreatic ductal adenocarcinoma is still highly lethal with five-year survival rate just around 5–7% and one-year survival is achieved in less than 20% of cases, reflecting the aggressive metastatic spread of PDAC and the lack of effective and reliable biomarkers for early diagnosis [2].

© Springer Nature Switzerland AG 2018
D. Stoyanov et al. (Eds.): POCUS 2018/BIVPCS 2018/CuRIOUS 2018/CPM 2018,
LNCS 11042, pp. 193–201, 2018.
https://doi.org/10.1007/978-3-030-01045-4_24

Therefore, there is an important need for development of novel and effective strategies for PDAC early detection and therapy.

Molecular techniques and imaging techniques have been developed for the diagnose and prognosis. Recent studies have utilized deep and targeted genomic analysis techniques to study pancreatic cancer [7]. These molecular techniques have been successful in characterizing gene-expression signatures in cancer cell and the molecular landscape of PDAC. But molecular techniques may not be able to sufficiently capture the heterogeneous nature of PDAC in vivo. While imaging techniques, especially computed tomography (CT) scan accompanied by three-dimensional (3D) reconstruction, are widely used for preoperative staging of PDAC [8,9]. Imaging techniques can provide quantitative phenotypic features to reveal the characteristics of tumors. Other clinical variables can also serve as reliable prognostic biomarkers. For example, CA19-9 levels evaluation is recommended to correctly stage PDAC, assess the response to therapy [3].

Prognostic models for the prediction of overall survival of PDAC is of vital importance because it can serve to predict the biological aggressiveness of this cancer and evaluate the patient outcome. Survival analysis, originated from clinical research, establishes a connection between covariates and the time of an event. It differs from traditional regression by the fact that parts of the training data can only be partially observed due to patient's dropout and study's limited time. By fitting the survival function and hazard function using covariates in a regression models, we can predict the prognosis of patients.

In this paper, we developed a prognostic model to predict overall survival based on predictors derived from contrast-enhanced pancreas CT scans and patient's clinical variables.

2   Method

2.1   Image Acquisition

The image dataset used in paper comes from the MICCAI 2018 computational precision medicine challenge, which focuses on the quantitative assessment of pancreas cancer. This dataset consists of a consecutive series of 212 patients undergoing pancreas resection at Memorial Sloan Kettering Cancer Center with clinical variables and high-quality annotated CT imaging. In which 159 portal venous phase CT images of the pancreas parenchyma and tumor in MetaImage (MHD) format are provided as a "training set". These images are fully anonymized, with expert radiologist segmented tumors and liver parenchyma to eliminate segmentation-related uncertainty. In addition to the image data, the training set includes a data dictionary describing the clinical variables and a list of the variables for each patient, including preoperative CA 19-9 and neoadjuvant chemotherapy.

2.2   Data Processing

Since gray values of CT scans reflect absolute world values (HU) and should be comparable between scanners, we don't perform intensity normalization on the

CT images. For the missing entries in preoperative CA 19-9, we fill the holes with the median value.

2.3   Image Analysis

We extraction of radiomics features from medical imaging to serve as events/covariates for survival analysis. For each CT scan, we extract features in three categories: first order statistics, shape-based features and texture features. In addition, we applied Laplacian of Gaussian and Wavelet filter to images, then extract features based on the filtered image. Each feature is extract from two kinds of region of interest (ROI), the first one is segmented tumor region by experts; the another one is drawn to encompass all pancreas region based on intensity values.

We also applied feature extraction on Wavelet filtered and Laplacian of Gaussian filtered images in addition to the original images. The Wavelet filtering yields 8 decompositions per level, which include all possible combinations of applying either a High or a Low pass filter in each of the three dimensions. The LoG filter enhances the edge by emphasizing areas of gray level change. Sigma value in LoG filter defines how coarse the emphasized texture should be. We extracted features from LoG filtered images with sigma value equals 1.0, 2.0, 3.0, 4.0, 5.0 respectively.

In total, we extracted 2436 features from each CT image. The features were extracted using custom code and *Pyradiomics* toolbox [4].

First Order Statistics. We extracted 19 features for first order statistics, which are described as follows.

Basic Features. For basic first order statistics, we extract the maximum intensity, minimum intensity, mean, median, 10th percentile, 90th percentile, standard deviation, variance of intensity value in ROI.

Energy. Energy is a measure of the magnitude of voxel values in an image. A larger values implies a greater sum of the squares of these values.

$$energy = \sum_{i=1}^{N_p} (\mathbf{X}(i))^2 \tag{1}$$

Total Energy. Total Energy is the value of Energy feature scaled by the volume of the voxel.

$$total\ energy = V_{voxel} \sum_{i=1}^{N_p} (\mathbf{X}(i) + c)^2 \tag{2}$$

Entropy. Entropy specifies the uncertainty/randomness in the image values. It measures the average amount of information required to encode the image values.

$$entropy = -\sum_{i=1}^{N_g} p(i) \log_2 \left(p(i) + \epsilon\right) \tag{3}$$

where ϵ is an arbitrarily small positive number.

Interquartile Range

$$interquartile\ range = \mathbf{P}_{75} - \mathbf{P}_{25} \tag{4}$$

where $\mathbf{P}_{25}$ and $\mathbf{P}_{75}$ are the 25th and 75th percentile of the gray level array, respectively.

Range

$$range = \max(\mathbf{X}) - \min(\mathbf{X}) \tag{5}$$

Mean Absolute Deviation (MAD)

$$MAD = \frac{1}{N_p} \sum_{i=1}^{N_p} |\mathbf{X}(i) - \bar{X}| \tag{6}$$

Mean Absolute Deviation is the mean distance of all intensity values from the Mean Value of the image array.

Robust Mean Absolute Deviation (rMAD)

$$rMAD = \frac{1}{N_{10-90}} \sum_{i=1}^{N_{10-90}} |\mathbf{X}_{10-90}(i) - \bar{X}_{10-90}| \tag{7}$$

Robust Mean Absolute Deviation is the mean distance of all intensity values from the Mean Value calculated on the subset of image array with gray levels in between, or equal to the 10th and 90th percentile.

Root Mean Squared (RMS)

$$RMS = \sqrt{\frac{1}{N_p} \sum_{i=1}^{N_p} (\mathbf{X}(i) + c)^2} \tag{8}$$

RMS is the square-root of the mean of all the squared intensity values. It is another measure of the magnitude of the image values. This feature is volume-confounded, a larger value of c increases the effect of volume-confounding.

Skewness

$$skewness = \frac{\mu_3}{\sigma^3} = \frac{\frac{1}{N_p} \sum_{i=1}^{N_p} (\mathbf{X}(i) - \bar{X})^3}{\left(\sqrt{\frac{1}{N_p} \sum_{i=1}^{N_p} (\mathbf{X}(i) - \bar{X})^2}\right)^3} \tag{9}$$

Skewness measures the asymmetry of the distribution of values about the Mean value. Depending on where the tail is elongated and the mass of the distribution is concentrated, this value can be positive or negative.

Kurtosis

$$kurtosis = \frac{\mu_4}{\sigma^4} = \frac{\frac{1}{N_p} \sum_{i=1}^{N_p} (\mathbf{X}(i) - \bar{X})^4}{\left(\frac{1}{N_p} \sum_{i=1}^{N_p} (\mathbf{X}(i) - \bar{X})^2\right)^2} \tag{10}$$

Kurtosis is a measure of the 'peakedness' of the distribution of values in the image ROI. A higher kurtosis implies that the mass of the distribution is concentrated towards the tail(s) rather than towards the mean. A lower kurtosis implies the reverse: that the mass of the distribution is concentrated towards a spike near the Mean value.

Uniformity

$$uniformity = \sum_{i=1}^{N_g} p(i)^2 \tag{11}$$

Uniformity is a measure of the sum of the squares of each intensity value. This is a measure of the homogeneity of the image array, where a greater uniformity implies a greater homogeneity or a smaller range of discrete intensity values.

2.4 Shape Features

We extracted 14 features to characterize the shape of ROI, which are described as follows.

Basic Features. For basic shape features, we extract volume, surface area, surface area to volume ratio, maximum 3D diameter, maximum 2D diameter for axial, coronal and sagittal plane respectively, major axis length, minor axis length and least axis length in ROI.

Sphericity

$$sphericity = \frac{\sqrt[3]{36\pi V^2}}{A} \tag{12}$$

Sphericity is a measure of the roundness of the shape of the tumor region relative to a sphere. It is a dimensionless measure, independent of scale and orientation. The value of 1 indicates a perfect sphere.

Spherical Disproportion

$$spherical\ disproportion = \frac{A}{4\pi R^2} = \frac{A}{\sqrt[3]{36\pi V^2}} \tag{13}$$

where R is the radius of a sphere with the same volume as the tumor, and equal to $\sqrt[3]{\frac{3V}{4\pi}}$.

Elongation

$$elongation = \sqrt{\frac{\lambda_{\text{minor}}}{\lambda_{\text{major}}}} \tag{14}$$

where λ_{major} and λ_{minor} are the lengths of the largest and second largest principal component axes.

Flatness

$$flatness = \sqrt{\frac{\lambda_{\text{least}}}{\lambda_{\text{major}}}} \tag{15}$$

where λ_{major} and λ_{least} are the lengths of the largest and smallest principal component axes.

2.5   Texture Features

We also extracted texture features using the standard pipeline of *Pyradiomics* toolbox, including 22 grey level co-occurrence matrix (GLCM) features, 16 gray level run length matrix (GLRLM) features, 16 Grey level size zone matrix (GLSZM) features, five neigbouring gray tone difference matrix (NGTDM) features and 14 gray level dependence matrix (GLDM) Features. Due to the page limitation we don't present the full list here, it can be found at https://pyradiomics.readthedocs.io/en/latest/features.html#module-radiomics.glcm

2.6   Survival Analysis

Feature Selection. Since the number of covariates is large relative to the number of observations, we performed feature selection remove the redundant or irrelevant features we extracted, as well as to reduce overfitting in model. More specifically, we fit a Cox model to each variable individually and record the c-index on the training set.

Next, we want to build a parsimonious model by excluding irrelevant features. We use the top ranking features as described above. By experimenting with five-fold cross-validation on the training set, we determined the number of features to use.

Survival Prediction. In order to perform accurate and robust prediction of the overall survival predication of patients' survival, we utilize gradient boosting with component-wise Cox's proportional hazards model as base learner [5].

We denotes D_i as the time from disease onset to death, and C_i as the potential time for patient i, $i = 1, \cdots, n$. Thus the observed survival time is $T_i = \min\{D_i, C_j\}$, and the death indicator is given by $\delta_i = I(D_i \leq C_i)$. Let $X_i = (X_{i1}, \cdots, X_{ip})^T$ be a p-dimensional covariate vector which contains all features selected for the ith patient. We assume that, conditional on X_i, D_i is independently censored by C_i. Then the death hazard can be modeled as

$$\lambda_i(t|X_i) = \lim_{dt \to 0} \frac{1}{dt} \Pr(t \leq D_i < t + dt | D_i \geq t, X_i) = \lambda_0(t) \exp(X_i^T \beta) \tag{16}$$

where $\lambda_0(t)$ denotes the baseline Coxs proportional hazards function. $\beta = (\beta_1, \cdots, \beta_p)$ is the vector of parameters. The corresponding log-partial likelihood is given by

$$(\beta) = \sum_{i=1}^{n} \delta_i \left[X_i^T \beta - \log\{ \sum_{\ell \in R_i} \exp(X_\ell^T \beta) \} \right] \tag{17}$$

The idea of gradient boosting is to pursue iterative steepest ascent of the log likelihood function. At each step, given the current estimate of β, say $\hat{\beta}$, let $\hat{\eta} = X^T \hat{\beta}$. The algorithm computes the gradient of the log-partial likelihood with respect to η_i, the ith component of η,

$$U_i = \frac{\delta}{\delta \eta_i} l_n(\eta)|_{\eta=\hat{\eta}} = \delta_i - \sum_{\ell=1}^{n} \frac{\delta_\ell I(T_i \geq T_\ell) \exp(\hat{\eta}_i)}{\sum_{k=1}^{n} I(T_k \geq T_\ell) \exp(\hat{\eta}_k)} \tag{18}$$

A component-wise algorithm can be implemented by restricting the search direction to be component-wise. For example, fit component-wise model

$$\tilde{\beta}_j = \arg\min_{\beta_j} \frac{1}{n} \sum_{i=1}^{n} (U_i - X_{ij} \tilde{\beta}_j)^2 \tag{19}$$

for $j = 1, \cdots, p$, compute

$$j^* = \arg\min_{1 \leq j \leq p} \frac{1}{n} \sum_{i=1}^{n} (U_i - X_{ij} \tilde{\beta}_j)^2 \tag{20}$$

and update $\hat{\beta}_{j*} = \hat{\beta}_{j*} + v\tilde{\beta}_{j*}$ until stop criteria is reaches. Here v denotes the learning rate. In our model, we set learning rate to 0.1 and number of boosting stages to 100.

3   Result

Based on the methods described above, we performed feature extraction, feature selection and survival prediction. For feature extraction, we extracted 2438 features per case, including 2436 image features and 2 clinical covariates. For feature selection, we fitted a Cox model to each variable individually and record the c-index on the training set, and used five-fold cross-validation on the training set to the number of features to use. In the end, we selected the following 16 features (Table 1):

Table 1. Selected most predicative features

Feature	Score
log-sigma-5-0-mm-3D_glszm_LargeAreaLowGrayLevelEmphasis_tumor	0.577367
wavelet-LLH_firstorder_RootMeanSquared_tumor	0.577107
log-sigma-5-0-mm-3D_glcm_Correlation_tumor	0.574764
original_shape_Maximum2DDiameterColumn_tumor	0.574503
log-sigma-3-0-mm-3D_glszm_ZoneEntropy_tumor	0.573201
wavelet-LHH_glszm_GrayLevelNonUniformity_tumor	0.568081
wavelet-LLH_glszm_GrayLevelNonUniformity_tumor	0.567300
wavelet-HLH_firstorder_Skewness_tumor	0.566519
log-sigma-5-0-mm-3D_glcm_Idmn_tumor	0.565825
log-sigma-5-0-mm-3D_glcm_Imc2_tumor	0.564523
wavelet-LHL_glszm_GrayLevelNonUniformity_tumor	0.564263
wavelet-HHL_glszm_LargeAreaHighGrayLevelEmphasis_tumor	0.563569
original_shape_Maximum2DDiameterSlice_tumor	0.563221
log-sigma-4-0-mm-3D_glcm_Correlation_tumor	0.562787
log-sigma-5-0-mm-3D_glcm_Imc1_tumor	0.562354
wavelet-HHL_gldm_SmallDependenceLowGrayLevelEmphasis_tumor	0.562267

Finally, we evaluate the performance of our model by predicting overall survival on training set based on predictors and calculated the concordance index. The experiments were done in five-fold cross-validation. We achieves the mean concordance index of 0.7016.

4   Discussion

In this paper, we developed a prognostic model to predict overall survival based on predictors derived from contrast-enhanced pancreas CT scans and patient clinical variables. We extracted radiomics features from CT scans, and fitted a Cox model to each variable individually to select the most predictive features. Finally, we use gradient boosting with component-wise Cox's proportional hazards model to predict the overall survival of patients. Our model achieves mean concordance index of 0.7016 using five-fold validation on training set. In the future, we will explore more possibilities of feature selection and survival predication methods to improve the performance of our model.

References

1. Adamska, A., Domenichini, A., Falasca, M.: Pancreatic ductal adenocarcinoma: current and evolving therapies. Int. J. Mol. Sci. **18**(7), 1338 (2017)
2. Brennan, M.F., Kattan, M.W., Klimstra, D., Conlon, K.: Prognostic nomogram for patients undergoing resection for adenocarcinoma of the pancreas. Ann. Surg. **240**(2), 293 (2004)
3. Distler, M., Pilarsky, E., Kersting, S., Grützmann, R.: Preoperative CEA and CA 19–9 are prognostic markers for survival after curative resection for ductal adenocarcinoma of the pancreas-a retrospective tumor marker prognostic study. Int. J. Surg. **11**(10), 1067–1072 (2013)
4. van Griethuysen, J.J., et al.: Computational radiomics system to decode the radiographic phenotype. Cancer Res. **77**(21), e104–e107 (2017)
5. He, K., et al.: Component-wise gradient boosting and false discovery control in survival analysis with high-dimensional covariates. Bioinformatics **32**(1), 50–57 (2015)
6. Siegel, R.L., Miller, K.D., Jemal, A.: Cancer statistics, 2017. CA: A Cancer J. Clin. **67**(1), 7–30 (2017). https://doi.org/10.3322/caac.21387
7. Oldfield, L.E., Connor, A.A., Gallinger, S.: Molecular events in the natural history of pancreatic cancer. Trends Cancer **3**(5), 336–346 (2017)
8. Rangarajan, V.: Three dimensional (3D) CT reconstruction in cancer imaging. Indian J. Med. Res. **137**(1), 10–11 (2013)
9. Zhu, L., et al.: CT imaging biomarkers predict clinical outcomes after pancreatic cancer surgery. Medicine **95**(5), e2664 (2016)

Author Index

Printed in the United States
by Baker & Taylor Publisher Services